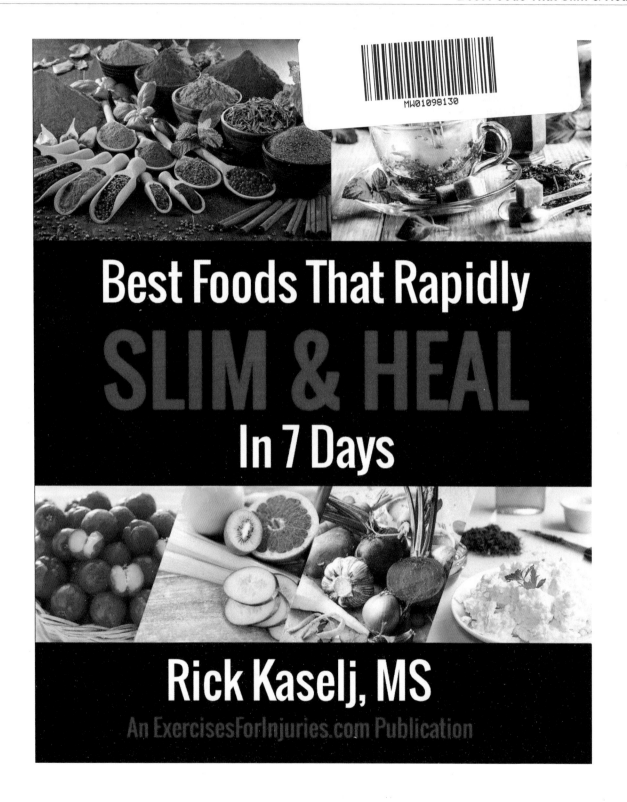

Best Foods That Rapidly

SLIM & HEAL

In 7 Days

Rick Kaselj, MS

An ExercisesForInjuries.com Publication

Rick Kaselj, MS, BSc, PK, CES
ExercisesForInjuries.com

Table of Contents

Title:
Best Foods that Rapidly Slim & Heal in 7 Days

Edition:
2nd Edition (January 2017)
1st Edition (July 2015)

Authors:
Kaselj, Rick

Keywords:
slimming foods, healing foods, muscle pain foods

Published by:

RK Exercises For Injuries
Suite #2289 - 3151 Lakeshore Rd
Kelowna, BC V1W 3S9
Canada
E-mail: support@ExercisesForInjuries.com
Webpage: www.ExercisesForInjuries.com

Phone: (888) 291-2430
Fax: (888) 291-2430

ISBN-13: 978-1543004304

ISBN-10: 154300430X

Rick Kaselj, MS, BSc, PK, CES
ExercisesForInjuries.com

Disclaimer

Best Foods that Rapidly Slim & Heal in 7 Days is primarily an educational resource and is not intended to take the place of the advice and recommendations of a physician. If you suspect your client has a health problem, please have him or her seek the services of a physician or healthcare professional.

The author has checked with sources believed to be reliable in his effort to provide information that is complete and generally in accord with the standards accepted at the time of publication. The information was accurate to the best of his knowledge. It is presented AS IS.

However, health nutrition is an ever-changing science. As new research and clinical experience broaden our knowledge, changes in diet and nutrition recommendations are inevitable. In view of the possibility of human error or changes in health nutrition, neither the author nor any other party who has been involved in the preparation or publication of this work warrants that the information contained herein is in every respect accurate or complete, and they are not responsible for any errors or omissions or for the results obtained from the use of such information. Readers are encouraged to confirm the information contained herein with other sources.

Legal Notice

Feel free to take your personal printed copy and share it with your family, friends and colleagues. Everyone's health will improve if we all learn and educate each other on how to maintain a healthy and active lifestyle.

If you received this as an e-book, please do not forward it on. Writing is how I make a living. Unauthorized distribution constitutes theft of my intellectual property. This will lead to felony charges, fines, possible prison time and bad karma. Just to be clear, you may NOT edit this document, extract from it, change the contents or offer it for sale in any way shape or form.

Any trademarks used in this book are the property of their respective owners.

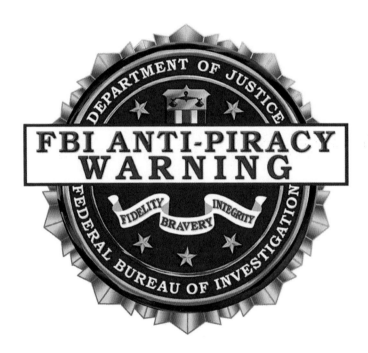

Rick Kaselj, MS, BSc, PK, CES
ExercisesForInjuries.com

Preface

Thank you for supporting one of my dreams!

I have always dreamed of being a writer. The book you are reading is one of those writing dreams coming true. I hope you take from it as much as I have gotten out of its research and production.

Pass this Book On

Feel free to take your personal printed copy and share it with your family, friends and colleagues. Everyone's health will improve if we all learn and educate each other on how to maintain a healthy and active lifestyle. If you received this as an e-book, please do not forward it on. Writing is how I make a living. Unauthorized distribution constitutes theft of my intellectual property.

Guarantee

My passion is to help people achieve a healthy and happy life. If this book does not help you, does not meet your expectations or is not of value to you, I will give you your money back. Please contact me via e-mail at support@ExercisesForInjuries.com and I will refund your money.

Contact Me

Please let me know what you think of this book. Visit www.ExercisesForInjuries.com or email me at support@ExercisesForInjuries.com. Your feedback and ideas will help with the content of future editions and books.

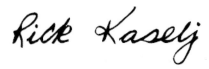

Rick Kaselj, MS, BSc, PK, CES
ExercisesForInjuries.com

Which Foods Can Slim, Trim, & Ease Joint and Muscle Pain

You've probably already heard that maintaining your health is about a lifestyle, not just a diet. And while that's absolutely correct, it doesn't take everyone's circumstances into consideration. The journey of a healthy lifestyle may start with a strict diet or an intense workout regimen. But what if an injury — whether inside or outside of a workout — occurs? This throws off half of that healthy lifestyle you had planned.

The truth is, the food we eat is what makes a majority of the difference when it comes to living healthy. You know what they say, "You are what you eat." Food is not only the fuel for your body, but it's also used to nourish your body and aid in healing. If you put good things in, you're going to get good results. In this book, you'll find out how different types of food — including vegetables, roots, berries, other fruits, and even herbs and spices — can slim and trim the body, as well as ease joint and muscle pain to keep your healthy journey right on track.

#1 - Vegetables

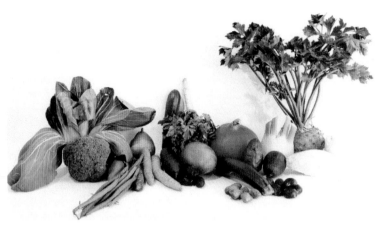

Vegetables are probably the first food item you think of when it's time to slim down and get healthy. And while no vegetable is bad for you, some of them are much healthier than others.

Slice up a cucumber and toss it on your next salad or as a snack between meals. Cucumber is 95% water, which works to flush out toxins and waste from the body. Since cucumbers are also rich in fiber, they work to make you feel full and control hunger cravings.

Lately, kale seems to be the popular vegetable in the garden, but not without good reason. Kale is a great source of fiber, keeping you full longer. Kale also delivers hefty servings of vitamin A and even calcium. For weight loss, include kale in your daily diet.

Aside from kale, arugula is a great green to add to your salads. This green contains protein (two cups of the stuff has 1 gram of protein), which will nourish and fill the body. It also contains vitamin A, vitamin K, vitamin C, folate, and even calcium.

Bell Peppers are a great, versatile vegetable you can have as a snack or as part of a meal. While they are filling, and contain lots of water, they are also full of vitamins, including vitamin A and C. They are also good for the joints, as they have anti-inflammatory properties and can offer pain relief.

Like kale, broccoli also contains lots of vitamins, as well as protein (more protein than kale per serving). It's a great food to eat for weight loss purposes, but also improves bone health and reduces inflammation.

And last but not least, Shiitake Mushrooms aren't necessarily known for their slimming properties, but they are a great food to add to your regular diet because they provide the body with iron and antioxidants, and are good for the cardiovascular system.

Rick Kaselj, MS, BSc, PK, CES
ExercisesForInjuries.com

#2 - Roots & Bulbs

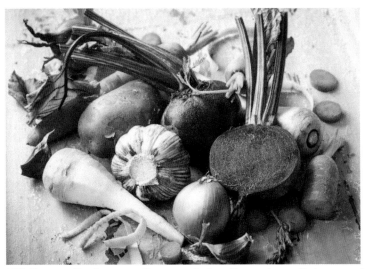

Most roots and bulbs are going to add lots of flavor to your dishes, but you can also add extra nutrients to give your body some benefits.

Adding onions to a dish is a great way to add flavor without adding sodium. Onions have high levels of antioxidants and promote heart health. They are also high in ohenolics and flavonoids. Phenolics and flavonoids help prevent cancer by cleaning up cell-damaging free radicals.

While garlic is mostly used for flavoring, it has a history of being used for its multitude of health benefits. While low in calories, garlic contains high amounts of vitamin C, vitamin B6, and manganese. Interestingly, garlic was one of the earliest forms of performance enhancement, although various results have been found.

Ginger is often known for its ability to settle an upset stomach, but it has other health benefits too. Ginger reduces inflammation, promotes circulation, and reduces pain.

#3 - Berries

Every single berry has great health benefits. When shopping for berries, keep this in mind; the darker the berry, the greater the benefits. Berries that are rich in color are also packed with nutrients and antioxidants that do the body wonders.

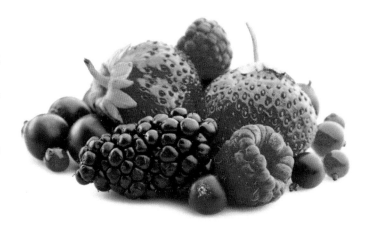

Blueberries have fat-burning properties and are known to assist in weight loss. They are also packed with vitamins, including vitamin C, E, and folate.

Rick Kaselj, MS, BSc, PK, CES
ExercisesForInjuries.com

#4 - Fruits

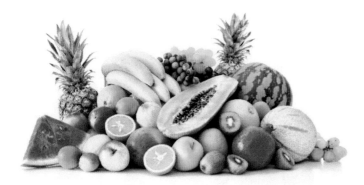

Berries aren't the only fruit that we can benefit from. Many other fruits, including citrus, can help you reach your fitness goals.

The saying may be true, "An apple a day keeps the doctor away!" An apple is home to soluble fiber, which is known to prevent blood sugar spikes that usually lead to unhealthy cravings. Make sure you go for an organic apple so that you can eat the peel, as that's where most of the nutrients live.

Pomegranate seeds are a fantastic source of antioxidants, and they also lower blood pressure and cholesterol. You may have to work a little to get the seeds out of a pomegranate, but you'll be rewarded greatly!

Eating cherries is one of the best ways you can reduce inflammation in the body, and can even aid in joint inflammation for those who have arthritis. Cherries are also a great way to prevent muscle damage. Enjoying cherries will also aid with muscle soreness post-workout.

Oranges contain high amounts of flavonoids, which have been known to have anti-inflammatory properties. They can also lower blood pressure and improve your overall heart health.

Grapefruit is a great choice for breakfast, or as a snack, because it has a compound known to lower insulin levels in the body and can lead to weight loss. Grapefruit is also home to enzymes and healthy carbohydrates that will keep you feeling full much longer.

Kiwi, the fuzzy fruit, is known for its slimming properties. It contains soluble, as well as insoluble fiber, which helps the body digest food. Kiwi also helps you feel full, which means you'll eat less and get slim! For best results, eat kiwi on an empty stomach.

#5 - Herbs

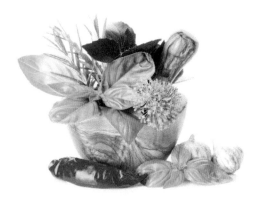

Much like roots and bulbs, most people think herbs are just for flavoring your food. And while they do add great flavor, many herbs have a history of healing the body.

Basil, a delicious addition to several Italian dishes, is also known to prevent inflammation and swelling. Basil is also very rich in antioxidants.

Cilantro is rich in vitamins and minerals, and may help to reduce "bad" cholesterol.

Parsley, often used as a garnish, flushes the kidneys and is known to help control blood pressure. Daily consumption relieves joint pain because of its anti-inflammatory properties.

Turmeric, a popular spice in curry dishes, contains high amounts of curcumin, which has powerful anti-inflammatory effects and serves as a strong antioxidant.

Wheat germ is home to lots of vitamin E, and aids sore muscles, as it has been shown to decrease exercise-induced muscle damage.

#6 - Other Foods

Surprisingly, cottage cheese is a great snack that will ease your post workout pain. The vitamin D in cottage cheese protects the body against joint pain, and its branched-chain amino acids protect muscle tissue from damage and soreness.

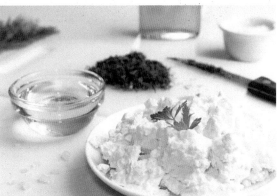

That extra virgin olive oil you've been cooking with and using as a salad dressing…it reduces pain the same way ibuprofen does. Who knew?

There are so many different options when it comes to eating a diet that's full of foods that will not only help slim and trim the body, but will also ease muscle and joint pain. Switch up your current diet and add in a few of the delicious foods from this list, and see what works for you. You just may find that living healthy is a little easier, and perhaps more delicious, than you originally thought.

Rick Kaselj, MS, BSc, PK, CES
ExercisesForInjuries.com

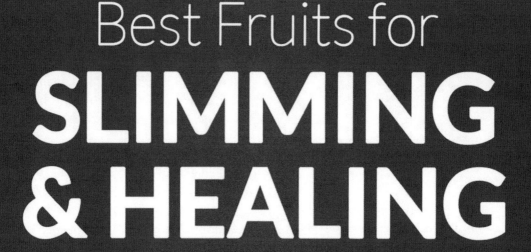

Best Fruits for
SLIMMING & HEALING

Rick Kaselj, MS | ExercisesForInjuries.com

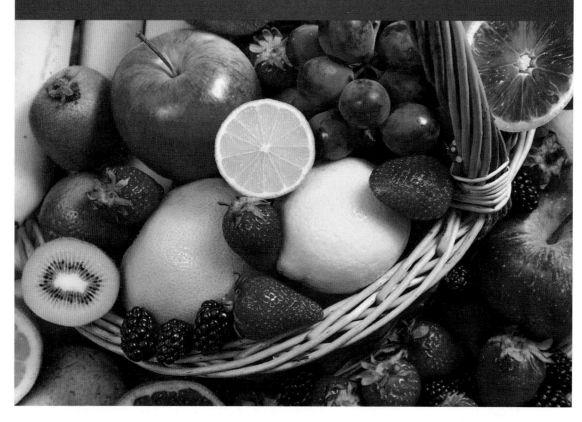

#1 – Oranges

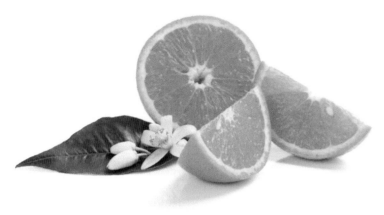

Oranges can be found almost anywhere. It is much better to eat fresh fruit than to depend on packaged fruit juices. Usually, oranges are sweet, which can help satisfy some of those cravings that occur when you are watching your weight. The calorie count for oranges is an AMAZING 47 calories for a 100g fresh orange. How does that sound for a new, slim you? Rich in vitamin C too, oranges are able to help the body heal from cuts and fight infections.

#2 - Grapefruit

High in fiber, grapefruits help you feel full! In addition, you consume about 74 calories in an average size grapefruit. That is really good news! Grapefruit helps to get your body's metabolism going and this in turn is GREAT FOR WEIGHT LOSS! The Journal for Medicinal Food published an article describing a research study which concluded that grapefruit is indeed able to lead to weight loss [3].

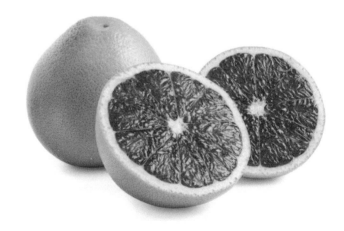

Rick Kaselj, MS, BSc, PK, CES
ExercisesForInjuries.com

#3 – Avocado

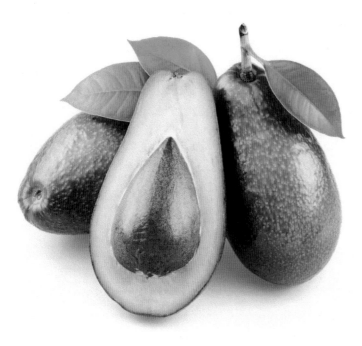

Seek out GOOD FATS such as avocados. You can lower cholesterol levels with avocados, and these monounsaturated fatty acid powerhouses are quite dense with nutrition [4]. These fats are also known as omega 9 fatty acids. Avocados help the body burn off excess fat and convert it to energy. This is definitely better than storing the fat in the body and packing on the pounds.

#4 - Pears

High in fiber content, pears can aid in digestion. You can count on pears to activate opportunities for weight loss, as the body uses all that fiber to push out unwanted waste content from the body. Doing so in a way that minimizes calorie intake while providing nutrition is SIMPLY WONDERFUL!

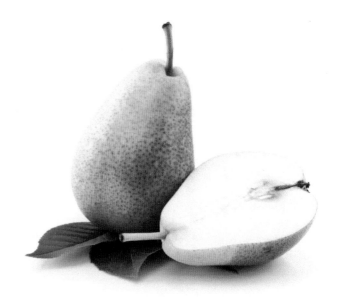

Rick Kaselj, MS, BSc, PK, CES
ExercisesForInjuries.com

#5 – Apples

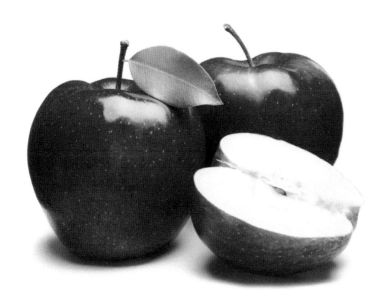

With well-known sayings such as, "an apple a day keeps the doctor away", apples have long been linked to a healthy lifestyle. Low in calorie count, high in fiber, and full of vitamin C and antioxidants, apples provide a great source of nutrition and opportunity for losing weight. An average size apple can contain about 50 calories. Hence, apples are a wonderful and EASY SNACK... you can enjoy an apple at any time of the day. Then sit back and enjoy a new slimmer and healthier you.

#6 – Coconut

Coconuts are simply one of nature's treasures. Yes, coconuts contain saturated fats, however these are not the fats that we should avoid. The fats in coconut do not remain in the body as fat! No... this is fat that is actually good for you to consume!! The fats in coconuts are triglyceride chains that are able to take the body's metabolic rate to a high level. And increasing your metabolism helps you LOSE WEIGHT! Coconuts are great as a snack and can be consumed as a fruit, coconut milk, and many other different ways.

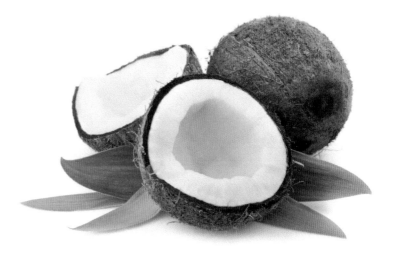

#7 – Lemons

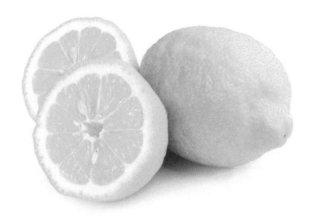

You may have seen folks putting lemons in their drinking water. Well ... there is a reason behind this and yes, it is related to weight loss. Lemons help to cleanse the body and while this cleansing is taking place, you are LOSING WEIGHT! How great!! Really... we should get our foods to work for us and not against us. Lemons are one of those fruits that you consume and know that it's helping your body to remove toxins and other wastes.

#8 – Papaya

Such a soft and smooth consistency and rich in color too... papayas are rich in carotenes. Yes, that rich orange color does come with something really good for you. Also, papaya contains flavonoids and vitamin C, which contribute to its healing properties. Papayas are also known to help foods transition through the body. In essence, eat papayas and your DIGESTIVE SYSTEM will thank you. Plus, you can lose weight too!

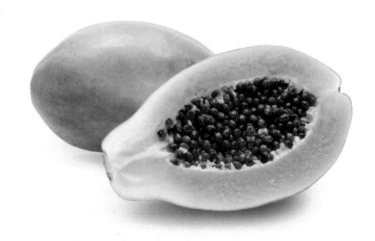

Rick Kaselj, MS, BSc, PK, CES
ExercisesForInjuries.com

#9 – Watermelon

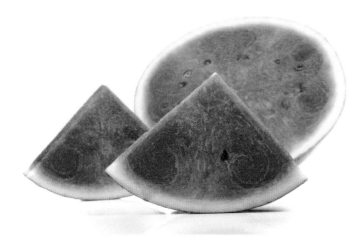

Watermelon contains arginine; an amino acid that helps to tackle fat. If you need a healthy snack, watermelon is a very good option. Great for weight loss, watermelons contain mostly... WATER! Well, there is no real surprise here as it can be seen in the name of this fruit. In fact, a watermelon is 90% water. What better weight loss technique can you find? Consuming 100g of watermelon results in a mere 30 calorie intake. With its high-water content, watermelons are also sure to keep you hydrated!

#10 – Mango

Mangoes are another great source of fiber and vitamin C. Full of vitamins A, B, E, K, and minerals such as calcium, be sure to eat mangoes when you need an energy boost. Fresh mangoes are great to have nearby. Mangoes have been identified as a way to fight obesity by reducing the fat in the body and getting blood sugar under control [5]. Consume in moderation though, because mangoes do contain more calories than some of the other fruits. However, there are still opportunities for slimming and healing with mangoes.

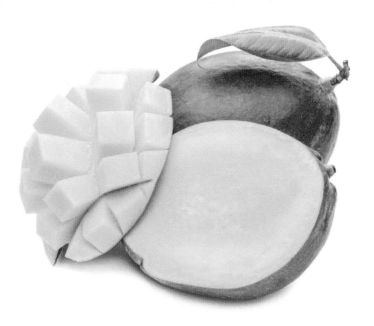

Rick Kaselj, MS, BSc, PK, CES
ExercisesForInjuries.com

#11 – Pineapples

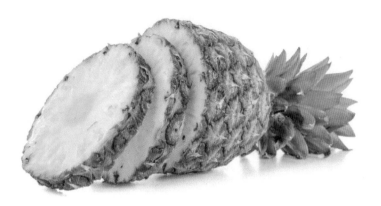

Just like watermelons, pineapples contain a lot of water (85%). This is important because water contains no calories, and if you are consuming no calories... guess what... YOU LOSE WEIGHT! Pineapples also provide you with essential vitamins, minerals and nutrients that the body needs to rejuvenate its cells and heal its tissues. The high water content in pineapples makes it easier to feel full and avoid overeating.

#12 – Kiwi

Kiwi fruits have an interesting appearance that takes nothing away from its ability to pump the body up with VITAMIN C. You need this vitamin, and being able to consume it from natural sources such as fruit is something you should not ignore. Kiwis are also low in calories, quite high in FIBER and help keep your appetite under control by making your tummy FEEL FULL.

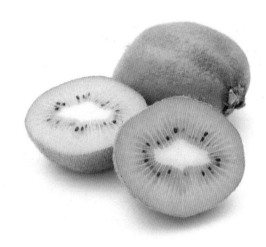

#13 – Bananas

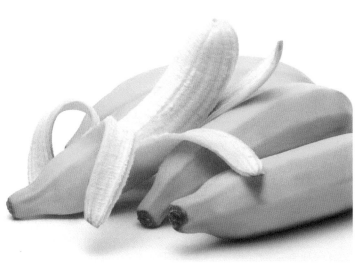

Although an average-sized banana contains a few more calories than other fruits, bananas are great for slimming and healing due to their ability to provide proper nourishment in comparison to snack options such as granola bars and fat-filled or sugar-filled choices. Greenish bananas have been known to contain high amounts of soluble starches which contribute to fat burning episodes within the body. Going to the gym for a workout?... bring along a banana for a NOURISHING post-workout snack!

#14 – Peaches

With just the right amount of sugar, peaches are just what you need to have a sweet fix while remaining on track with weight loss. Your body needs energy and peaches can provide this energy in a manner that is healthy! Don't seek ways to boost your energy that come from processed foods. You may get a short-term boost only to crash down! Focus on great sources of energy, like peaches and other fruits.

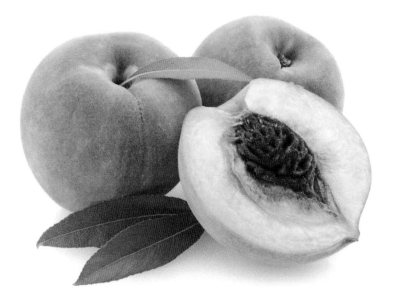

Rick Kaselj, MS, BSc, PK, CES
ExercisesForInjuries.com

#15 – Guava

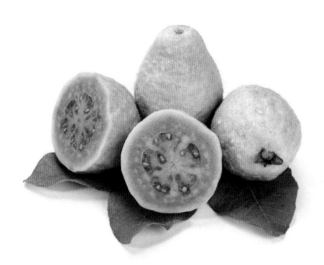

Lose weight by eating guava, which is high in fiber and has a low glycemic index. By eating guava, you'll reap the benefits of tidier bowel movements. Its rich fiber content can also make you feel full, thereby contributing to weight loss. According to the International Journal of Microbiology, guava also has antimicrobial effects, especially in terms of its leaves which have been found to possess the traits of a natural antimicrobial agent to fight infections [6]. This makes it great for healing and restoration of the body.

The great thing about fruits is that they hardly have any fat, and as a result are low in calories. It's worth the emphasis... so, let's say it again... FRUITS are practically FAT FREE. Considering the amount of other foods containing fat which are consumed regularly, it is easy to see why weight gain happens. However, by simply SWITCHING to a diet that includes more fruits, you can cut your CALORIE INTAKE tremendously and heal the body.

References

[1] Can eating fruits and vegetables help people to manage their weight?: http://www.cdc.gov/nccdphp/dnpa/nutrition/pdf/rtp_practitioner_10_07.pdf

[2] Children eating more fruit, but fruit and vegetable intake still too low: http://www.cdc.gov/media/releases/2014/p0805-fruits-vegetables.html

[3] The effects of grapefruit on weight and insulin resistance: relationship to the metabolic syndrome: http://www.ncbi.nlm.nih.gov/pubmed/16579728

[4] An avocado a day keeps the cardiologist away: http://news.psu.edu/story/339842/2015/01/07/research/avocado-day-keeps-cardiologist-away

[5] NSCI RESEARCH FINDS HEALTH BENEFITS IN MANGOS: http://humansciences.okstate.edu/nsci/index.php/component/content/article/1-latest/56-nsci-research-finds-health-benefits-in-mangos

[6] Antimicrobial Activities of Leaf Extracts of Guava: http://www.hindawi.com/journals/ijmicro/2013/746165/

Rick Kaselj, MS, BSc, PK, CES
ExercisesForInjuries.com

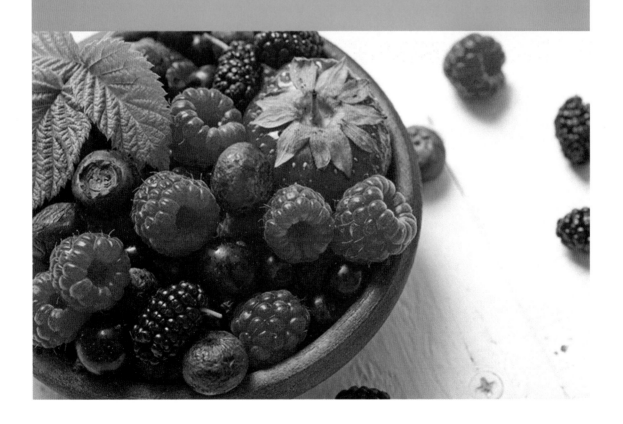

Best Berries for

SLIMMING & HEALING

Rick Kaselj, MS | ExercisesForInjuries.com

#1 – Blueberries

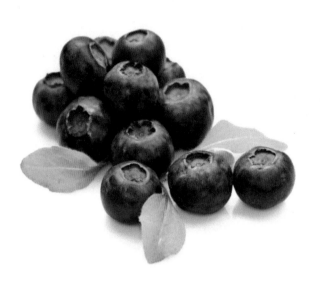

Blueberries sit on top of a powerhouse throne for their ability to provide the body with a SUPER HUGE dose of antioxidants. Their trademark deep blue color can add life to any dish and as most berries do, blueberries can add a touch of color to most foods. When the body is overrun by free radicals (that contribute to making us sick and generally unhealthy), blueberries come to the rescue every time by neutralizing these free radicals.

#2 - Goji Berries

It is difficult to miss the deep red color of these berries. There have been scientific linkages between goji berries and positive responses from cancer patients, including increased strength. There have also been studies done to show that goji berries have effects on macular characteristics and levels of antioxidant plasma as a result of the high antioxidant content of this berry [3].

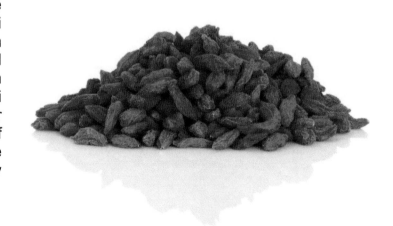

Rick Kaselj, MS, BSc, PK, CES
ExercisesForInjuries.com

#3 – Cherries

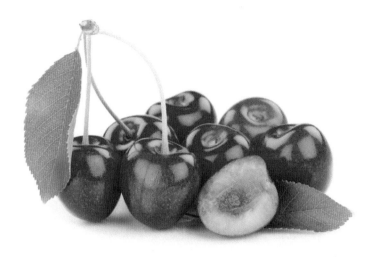

Simply beautiful to look at and delicious to eat, cherries are another antioxidant berry rich in flavonoids and anthocyanins, helping to rejuvenate tissues and promote cell health. There are a lot of research studies related to cherries and their impact on cancer [4]. Rich in melatonin, cherries cause you to relax and sleep better. Sleep can be a vital part of the healing process for your body. A Northumbria University research study found that cherries can reduce the effects of gout [5].

#4 – Pomegranates

There have been research studies regarding the status of pomegranates as nature's power fruit, and reports of this fruit's ability to treat various conditions, including mouth and gum diseases [6]. Quite the colorful fruit, pomegranates come in many varieties and can also be grown in many parts of the world. Research has also linked extracts from pomegranates to the selective inhibition of the growth of colon, lung, prostate and breast cancer [7].

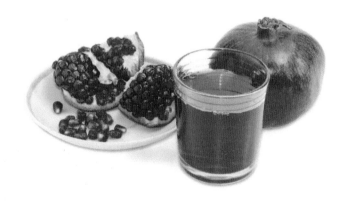

#5 – Strawberries

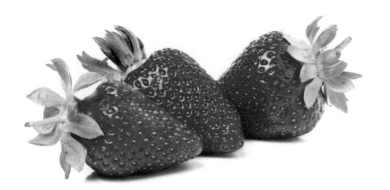

Another colorful and delicious berry, strawberries contain phenols which are able to boost our health and provide protection from the occurrence of disease. Throw some strawberries into your salads or cereals... or simply snack on them plain. You'll be glad you did.

#6 – Bilberries

What is a bilberry, anyway? While not the most well-known, bilberries certainly do not disappoint. One thing you may notice right away regarding bilberries is their size. These berries can be quite small, however their size does not take away from their ability to heal the body. Bilberries are rich in anthocyanidins antioxidants. When the body suffers from oxidation, such as the deterioration or degeneration of blood vessel lining or macular degeneration, bilberries are able to STEP UP and provide the

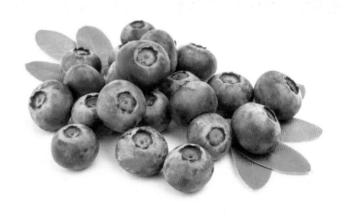

HEALING POWER required for repairing this issue. Some folks refer to bilberries as dyeberries, huckleberries, or wineberries.

Rick Kaselj, MS, BSc, PK, CES
ExercisesForInjuries.com

#7 – Acai Berries

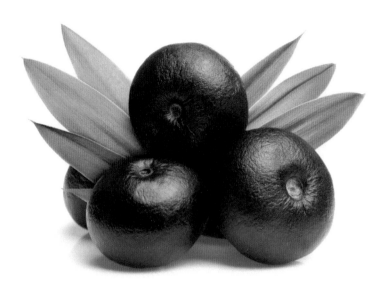

The acai berry is another strong contender in the world of POWERFUL ANTIOXIDANTS. Little was known about the acai berry until several years ago, but discovering this berry in the rainforests of the Amazon has resulted in the emergence of a food that has TWICE the anti-oxidant power of blueberries. This food is certainly becoming a king in the berry kingdom with regards to its antioxidant levels.

#8 – Blackberries

These berries are... well... black in color. NO surprise there! Blackberries contain vitamins E and C, which are great for fighting diseases. If you want HEALING, you'll want blackberries in your diet. You'll also find ellagic acid in blackberries to further enhance their disease fighting potential.

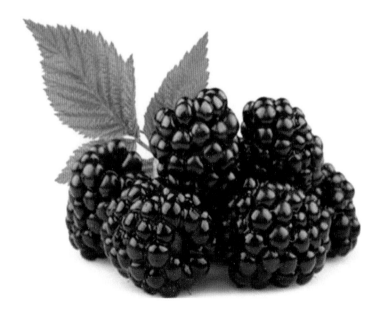

Rick Kaselj, MS, BSc, PK, CES
ExercisesForInjuries.com

#9 – Golden Berries

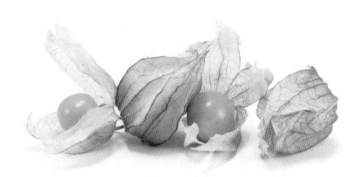

Known for their golden color, golden berries are a great source of vitamin B. They are rich in fiber too, helping you feel full and eat healthy! With golden berries as part of your diet, the body is able to regulate its metabolism more efficiently. You could mix these berries with other berries you are more familiar with for a tasty snack!

10 – Camu Camu Berries

Quite intriguing name, right? Yes, camu camu berries are great for keeping your skin looking youthful and healthy. Also, camu camu berries have been found to help the eyes and gums. Indeed, they do have a name that's quite catchy and pack a POWERFUL PUNCH in terms of their healing potential.

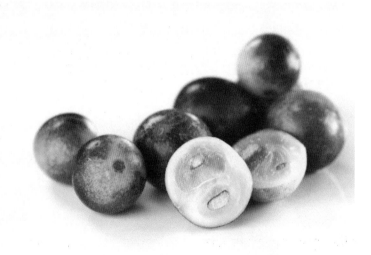

Rick Kaselj, MS, BSc, PK, CES
ExercisesForInjuries.com

#11 – Cranberries

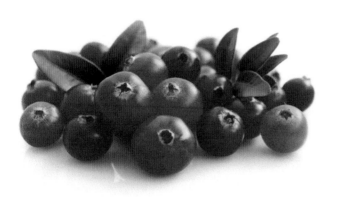

Great for fighting infections, cranberries have flavonoids that provide protection against urinary tract infections. These flavonoids are also known as proanthocyanidins. Cranberry juice, freshly squeezed, is a great alternative to sugary drinks and other less healthy options. You can do a lot for your waistline and health by simply making seemingly small choices, like adding these little berries to your diet.

#12 – Mulberries

One component of mulberries that makes it easy to consider this berry a 'MUST-HAVE', is polyphenols which keep the heart healthy. The healing power of mulberries also comes from its significant amounts of potassium, iron, magnesium, vitamin C and calcium. The vitamins aid the healing process in the body, while the calcium makes your bones stronger.

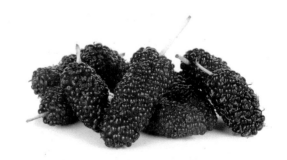

Rick Kaselj, MS, BSc, PK, CES
ExercisesForInjuries.com

#13 – Maqui Berries

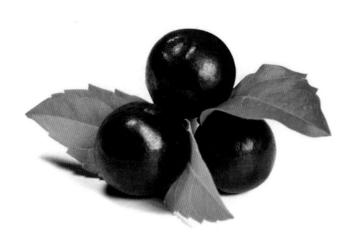

Perhaps you've not heard of maqui berries. Nevertheless, these berries are great for reducing inflammation and fighting fevers. High in flavonoids, maqui berries also keep the heart healthy and help to keep blood sugar levels within normal ranges.

#14 – Sea Buckthorn Berries

The sea buckthorn berry is nature's MULTI-VITAMIN. Quite the powerhouse with regards to your daily required vitamin intake, including vitamins C, E, K, A and the B complex vitamins. Did you ever imagine that such a seemingly simple food could contain such POWERFUL NUTRITION? Keep a bowl of sea buckthorn berries nearby!

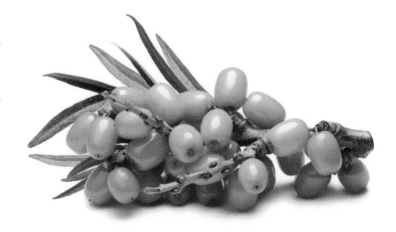

Rick Kaselj, MS, BSc, PK, CES
ExercisesForInjuries.com

#15 – Acerola Cherry

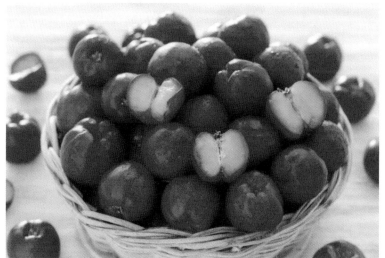

Acerola cherries are also referred to as Barbados cherries or simply as Acerola. Once you eat this cherry, prepare for a vitamin C party in your mouth! It's SUPER RICH in vitamin C. Acerola cherries can provide at least nine times more vitamin C than oranges. Can you imagine that?

#16 – Noni Berry

In the South Pacific tropics, noni berries can be easily sourced. Great for the digestive track, noni berries are known to take care of problems with the bowels and also soothe cramps or muscle spasms. Noni berries are also rich in vitamin C, vitamin B3, and some vitamin A. They also contain some calcium, which is great for STRENGTHENING BONES!! However, processing these berries, such as by squeezing out its juice, can result in a loss of some of these nutrients.

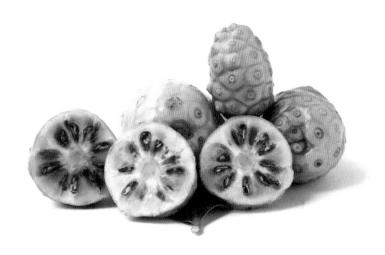

Rick Kaselj, MS, BSc, PK, CES
ExercisesForInjuries.com

#17 – Aronia – Black Chokeberry

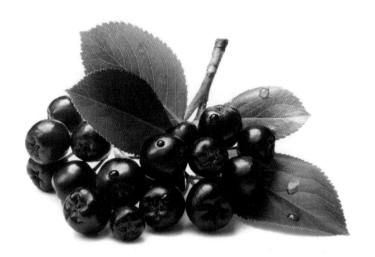

Don't let the name scare you away. The black chokeberry, or aronia berry, is similar to blueberries in size and contains large amounts of flavonoids. This berry gets its name from its powerful taste. Yes, certainly no mildness with the black chokeberry. Rather, you'll find this berry pungent with a biting feel as you eat it. It is still quite powerful in terms of its anthocyanins, vitamins and minerals. The aronia berry also contains antioxidants that provide great healing power.

#18 – Raspberry

These berries are extremely high in ellagic acid. Raspberries can also provide vitamin C, manganese, folic acid, copper and iron. How do raspberries help you lose weight? Their HIGH FIBER CONTENT! But, that's not all... Raspberries have a ketone compound that that has been linked to weight loss (however more research in this area is warranted). Research has also linked raspberries to the reduction of colorectal cancer tumors in mice [8].

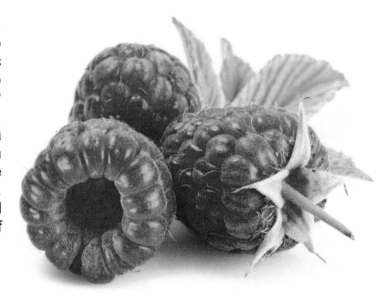

Rick Kaselj, MS, BSc, PK, CES
ExercisesForInjuries.com

Because of their high antioxidants, berries can help prevent diseases related to cell damage and oxidative stress that the body could be battling. Such high levels of antioxidants also aid in rejuvenation and could add a positive spin on the aging process. Now, WHO would NOT LIKE THAT?! Sometimes, we simply STICK WITH WHAT WE KNOW. For instance, oranges are typically the "go-to" fruit for vitamin C, but other fruits can be great too. So, if you have a cold or need some vitamin C, eat berries! Tap into any of the best berries for slimming and healing.

References

[1] Flavoniod-rich diet may reduce risk of type 2 diabetes: http://snowcrest.ca/category/healthy-living/

[2] What is a Flavonoid?: http://www.mnn.com/food/healthy-eating/stories/what-is-a-flavonoid

[3] Goji berry effects on macular characteristics and plasma antioxidant levels: http://www.ncbi.nlm.nih.gov/pubmed/21169874

[4] American Institute for Cancer Research– Foods that fight cancer Cherries: http://www.aicr.org/foods-that-fight-cancer/cherries.html

[5] Drinking Montmorency cherry concentrate reduces effects of gout: https://www.northumbria.ac.uk/about-us/news-events/news/2014/09/drinking-montmorency-cherry-concentrate-reduces-effects-of-gout/

[6] The Pomegranate: Nature's Power Fruit?: http://folk.uio.no/runeb/pdf filer/Logtin JNCI 2003 Pomegranates.pdf

[7] Cancer Chemoprevention by Pomegranate: Laboratory and Clinical Evidence: http://www.ncbi.nlm.nih.gov/pmc/articles/PMC2989797/

[8] Black Raspberries Help Prevent Colorectal Cancer in Mice: http://www.livescience.com/35123-black-raspberries-ward-off-colorectal-cancer-in-mice.html

Rick Kaselj, MS, BSc, PK, CES
ExercisesForInjuries.com

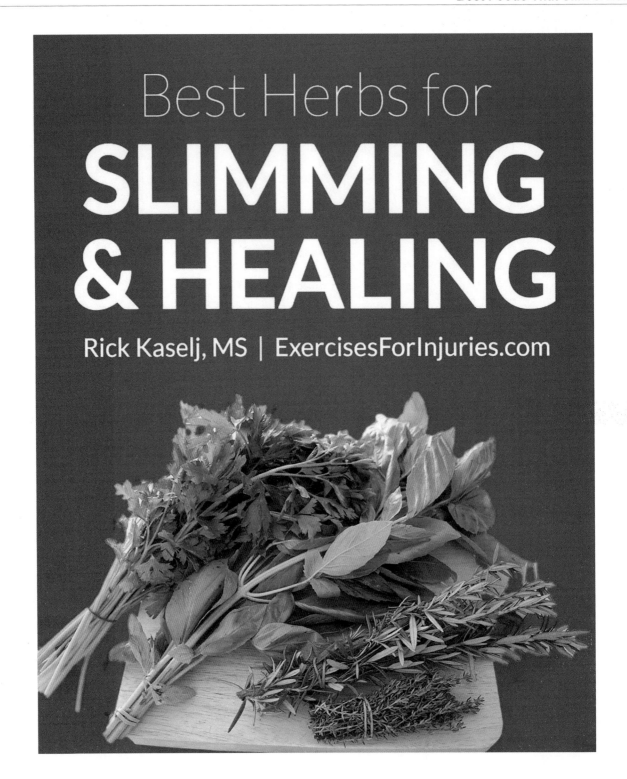

Best Herbs for
SLIMMING
& HEALING

Rick Kaselj, MS | ExercisesForInjuries.com

#1 – Rosemary

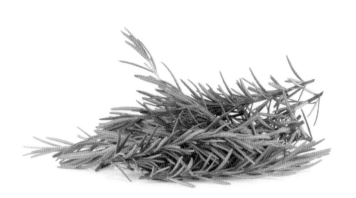

This herb has been linked to long-term memory... hmm, rosemary helps you remember! In a recent study conducted by Northumbria University, researchers reported that rosemary is connected to memory, increasing long-term memory and alertness by up to 75% [2]. Add this herb to meals and dishes, as it is low calorie and delicious. It is quite accessible too, making it very attractive for use in your kitchen!

#2 - Sage

Originating in the Mediterranean, sage is good for memory. It has a high antioxidant content, can tackle free radicals in the body, fight chronic diseases, and has been linked to possible treatments for Alzheimer's disease, high blood glucose and high cholesterol [3]. Other research studies specifically point to the use of sage as a natural way to prevent and cure illnesses like depression, diabetes, lupus, obesity, diabetes,

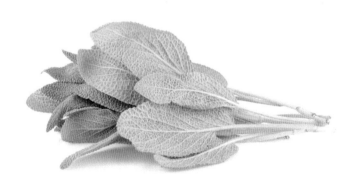

heart disease, cancer, autism and dementia [4]. Quite the list, right?!! Sage is indeed a powerful herb.

#3 – Oregano

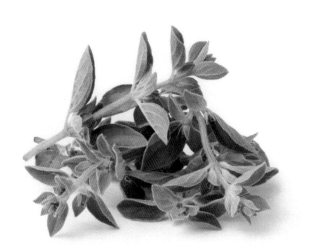

Packed with antifungal and antibacterial compounds, oregano can be used to treat yeast-based infections. Oil of Oregano has been called the "king of oils", and can be used to treat diabetes, allergies, lice, athlete's foot, colds, parasites, sores, ringworm and skin infections [4]. This is another powerful herb! Oregano can leave you feeling and looking healthy all over.

#4 – Basil

This is such an aromatic herb and used in many different types of cooking, such as Italian and Mediterranean foods. Sauces, salads, and salsa can all taste great with basil. Researchers' studies suggest that the basil herb can be used to fight chronic diseases, bacteria, and viruses [5]. Low calorie counts can also help with weight loss or maintenance. You are in good hands with this herb. Holy basil, is a variant of the basil family, can be used to treat episodes of high cholesterol. Other ailments that may benefit from the consumption of holy basil include diabetes, asthma, infections and pain.

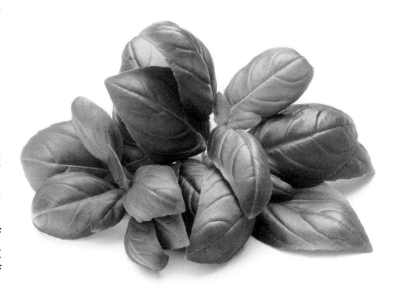

Rick Kaselj, MS, BSc, PK, CES
ExercisesForInjuries.com

#5 – Mint

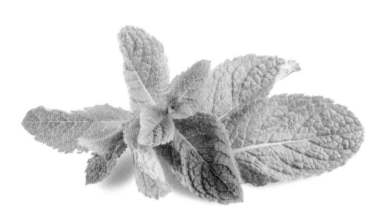

Now, who doesn't like mint? Add mint to salads, yogurt, as a side garnish, and much, much more! It's quite the versatile herb; readily available and user-friendly. It typically requires minimal chopping and is able to be tossed into foods within seconds. No hassle, no fuss! Medically, mint is associated with the treatment of IBS – irritable bowel syndrome and other digestive ailments. Specifically, peppermint has been shown to be quite effective for IBS [6].

#6 – Thyme

Easy to add to meals and great for the body too – thyme is quite the spice. There are essential thyme oils and fresh thyme versions. Thyme can be used for treating skin ailments such as acne, and it has been noted by the Society of General Microbiology that thyme could be more effective than prescription creams [7]. In addition, thyme oil suppresses inflammation [8]. It is another versatile herb and usually readily available in most grocery stores and farmers' markets. Thyme is a delightful tasting herb that can be used in many ways.

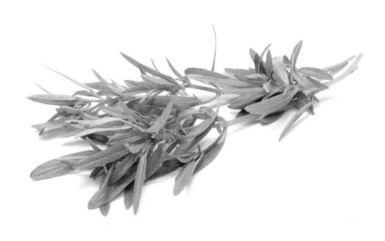

#7 – Ashwagandha

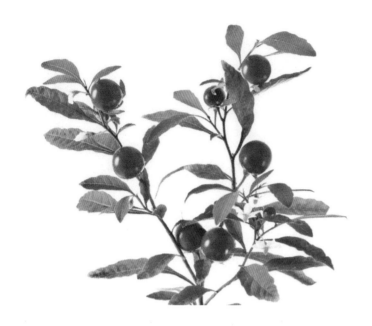

Names like this are quite the mouthful! But don't give up yet, even if the name may initially be difficult to pronounce. Ailments that the ashwagandha herb treats include inflammation, anxiety and high blood pressure. These can be really serious ailments and something that attention should be given to. Wouldn't you say that ashwagandha is looking very attractive right now?

#8 – Burdock

Although often considered a root, much of this plant is edible, including the root, leaves and seeds, making it quite the all-encompassing herb. It seems to HAVE IT ALL! An anti-inflammatory and antibacterial herb, this plant can fight bacterial infections and remove toxins. Burdock has therapeutic uses and although it has been used for centuries, the desire to research the herb and further understand its potential is becoming more rampant in research domains. It's good for your health and waistline.

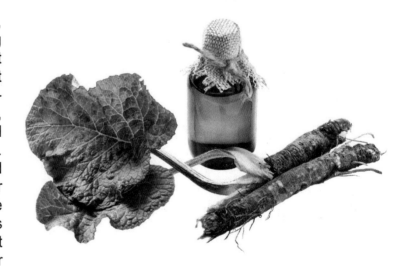

Rick Kaselj, MS, BSc, PK, CES
ExercisesForInjuries.com

#9 – Calendula

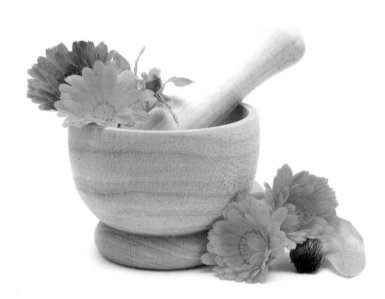

The bright yellow flowers are a distinguishing factor of this herb. It is useful for tackling ailments that affect the stomach, and has a rich antioxidant profile as well. You can fight inflammation and germs with this herb. In addition to treating stomach bugs, you can use calendula for the skin and to heal cuts. All around good for healing for your body, hold onto the anti-inflammatory, antiviral and anti-genotoxic properties of calendula.

#10 – Dandelion

Unfortunately, dandelions are considered a weed in some parts of the world. However, they can be quite the BENEFICIAL HERB. There have been connections between dandelions and the liver or kidney in terms of cleansing or using the herb as a diuretic. With minimal calories and healing potential, there is more to this herb that may meet the eye.

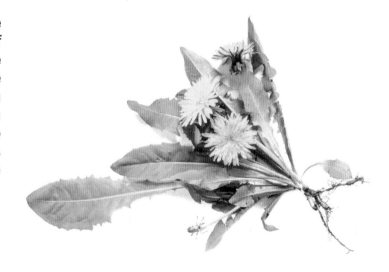

#11 – Lavender

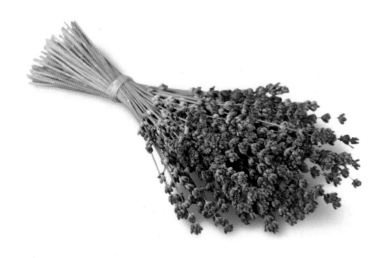

Soothing and calming... that's one way to describe lavender. You'll notice that lavender is used in many types of soaps and lotions for this very reason. Due to this calming effect, lavender can help people get to sleep easier and stay asleep throughout the night. It can also be used as a stress reliever during the day. How does this help slim and heal? Well... to heal, the body needs quality rest and limited stress. Lavender is also believed to reduce bloating.

#12 – Milk Thistle

This herb has a unique looking flower and is rich in antioxidants. Antioxidants can provide the body with healing support and tackle free radicals. In essence, antioxidants help keep us healthy. There are also other medical uses of milk thistle. Used for cancer treatment, milk thistle is undergoing studies to determine how it impacts delayed growth of cancerous tumors. Again, it's another low-calorie herb and good for keeping your weight at healthy levels.

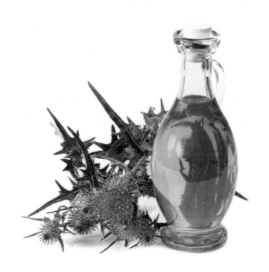

Rick Kaselj, MS, BSc, PK, CES
ExercisesForInjuries.com

#13 – Aloe Vera

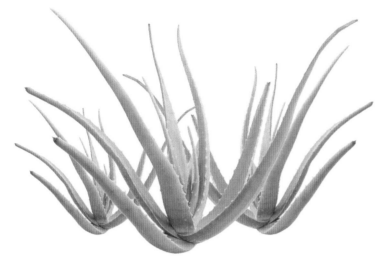

Many people grow this herb in their homes. You can use aloe vera for a multitude of purposes, both internally and externally. It can be used for cleaning the digestive system and for enhancing the digestive process. Have you seen aloe vera creams and ointments? It is great for the skin, helping to sooth sun burns, heal minor cuts and wounds, and reduce dry skin. It even helps to flush out toxins. So, keep your digestive tract healthy and nurture your skin with this herb!

#14 – Chickweed

Chickweed has been associated with weight loss. It may be consumed in many ways, including in raw form or cooked lightly. The University of Michigan Health System describes chickweed as being high in vitamin C and flavonoids, which enable its use as a skin irritation treatment [9]. Other skin conditions that chickweed can be used for include skin soreness, itching, insect bites and eczema.

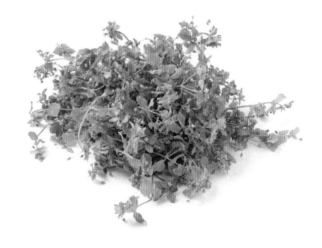

Rick Kaselj, MS, BSc, PK, CES
ExercisesForInjuries.com

#15 – Evening Primrose

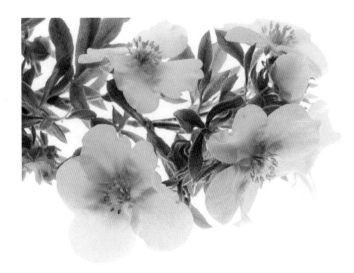

The evening primrose herb is another weight loss powerhouse that has a compound known as tryptophan. This herb can be taken daily and there are many evening primrose supplements that provide the same benefits.

#16 – Guggul

Maybe not a common name, guggul is popularly used in Ayurveda. It can be consumed regularly and is used to reduce and maintain a healthy weight. There have also been some linkages between guggul and the lowering of cholesterol levels. This is another herb in which further research is needed. However, you can enjoy its weight loss benefits as further details regarding other benefits of this herb emerge.

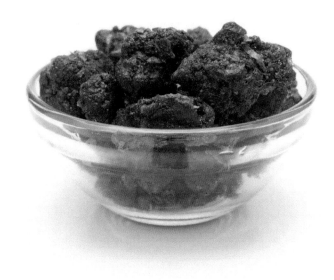

Rick Kaselj, MS, BSc, PK, CES
ExercisesForInjuries.com

#17 – Siberian Ginseng

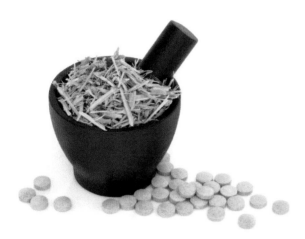

If you are craving sugar, Siberian ginseng may be just the thing you need to curb your appetite. This herb is a blood sugar regulator and helps to keep blood sugar levels stable. There are cautions to consider when using this herb, and individuals with high blood pressure need to discuss their condition with their doctor before using ginseng. Many people consume ginseng daily.

Herbs are well ... HERBS!! I mean, how much simpler can it get? These plants are really GOOD FOR YOU!! Herbs are rich in nutrients and low in calories. This double combination provides you with slimming potential and the ability to also dig into the deep, natural nutritional, medicinal reserves that these herbs have. So, what are you waiting for? Dive right in and discover the herbs around you. Use this list as a guide to a slimmer and healthy body!

References

[1] Use of Herbs Among Adults Based on Evidence-Based Indications: Findings From the National Health Interview Survey: http://www.ncbi.nlm.nih.gov/pmc/articles/PMC1964882/

[2] Why a whiff of rosemary does help you remember: http://www.dailymail.co.uk/health/article-2306078/Why-whiff-rosemary-does-help-remember.html

[3] What are the health benefits of sage?: http://www.medicalnewstoday.com/articles/266480.php

[4] Chemistry, Pharmacology, and Medicinal Property of Sage (*Salvia*) to Prevent and Cure Illnesses such as Obesity, Diabetes, Depression, Dementia, Lupus, Autism, Heart Disease, and Cancer: http://www.ncbi.nlm.nih.gov/pmc/articles/PMC4003706/

[5] From lab to lunch - Basil: http://www.precisionnutrition.com/wordpress/wp-content/uploads/2009/11/from-lab-to-lunch-basil.pdf

[6] How peppermint helps to relieve irritable bowel syndrome: http://www.sciencedaily.com/releases/2011/04/110419101234.htm

[7] Thyme may be better for acne than prescribed creams: http://www.sciencedaily.com/releases/2012/03/120327215951.htm

[8] Thyme oil can inhibit COX2 and suppress inflammation: http://www.sciencedaily.com/releases/2010/01/100113122306.htm

[9] University of Michigan Health System - Chickweed: http://www.uofmhealth.org/health-library/hn-2068006

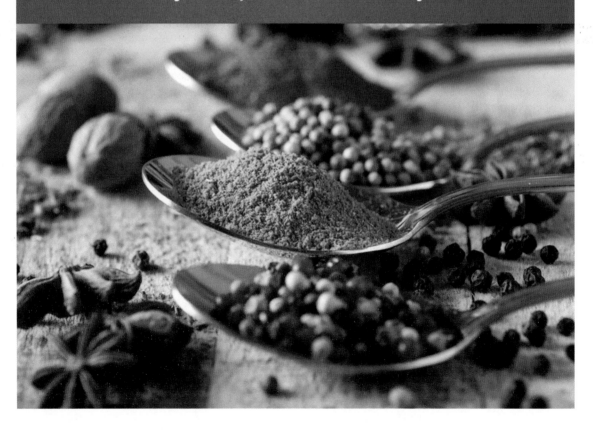

Best Spices for
SLIMMING
& HEALING

Rick Kaselj, MS | ExercisesForInjuries.com

Rick Kaselj, MS, BSc, PK, CES
ExercisesForInjuries.com

#1 – Garlic

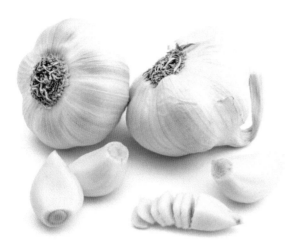

It's difficult to miss this spice! It has quite the unique taste and after-taste too. Hence, you may want to watch your daily garlic portions. Garlic does have many health benefits, including enabling the body to more efficiently metabolize fats and carbohydrates. Garlic may be crushed or chopped in fresh form, and added to dishes such as stews, sauces, rice and many other foods. You could also use the powdered form of this spice for that added kick to your meals.

#2 - Turmeric

An ancient spice more commonly found in India and Asia, turmeric is good for fighting inflammation, loosening stiff joints, and accelerating the wound healing process. A member of the ginger family, research has shown that turmeric provides antioxidants that can help minimize the appearance of free-radicals in the body.

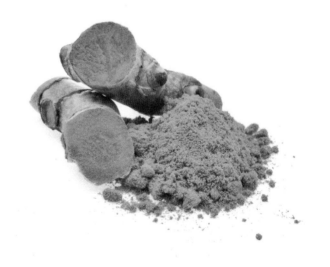

#3 – Cinnamon

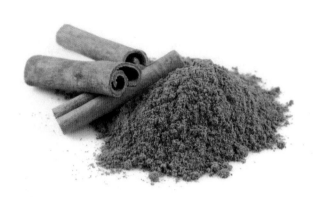

This spice can help to keep BLOOD SUGAR LEVELS under control. Eating cinnamon can also help control insulin levels, keeping you safe from the onset of diabetes. Cinnamon is quite tasty and used for adding flare to cereal or sprinkling on other foods. Many drinks are also made with cinnamon. Be creative and discover how to convert this spice option into one that WINS FOR YOU, all the time!

#4 – Saffron

Saffron research studies have been related to depression, macular conditions and degeneration, cancer, weight loss, Alzheimer disease, diabetes, anxiety and others. In terms of cancer research, studies related to animal models with cultures of human malignant cancer cells show that saffron is able to provide demonstrated anti-tumor and preventive cancer activities [2]. Weight loss and weight management have also been associated with saffron. One example of such

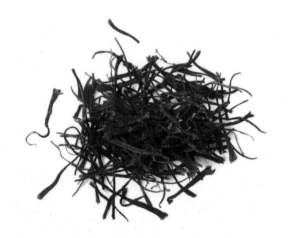

research was the positive impact of saffron on stress-induced anorexia in mice [3]. Cooking with saffron is quite the treat as well. Explore this spice today!

Rick Kaselj, MS, BSc, PK, CES
ExercisesForInjuries.com

#5 – Star Anise

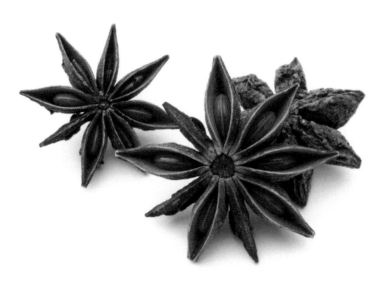

A good source of antioxidants, star anise can be quite the addition to your meals. This spice is known for its antifungal and antimycotoxigenic properties, and has been deemed a good exploratory source of newer and safer supplements [4]. Current research regarding star anise is looking very promising. Its antioxidant content alone is enough to warrant the use of this spice in your home. Next time you pass the spice section in the grocery store or market, add it to your shopping basket... and to your recipes!

#6 – Black Pepper

Although not the hottest pepper out there, black pepper does have a sufficient heat for most palettes. Black pepper can help you shed some pounds and even has healing potential. It tastes great added to many foods and burns calories too! What else could we ask for? We don't have to tell you that burning calories translates into weight loss. What you probably didn't know, is that it does so by using a process called thermogenesis in order to burn calories.

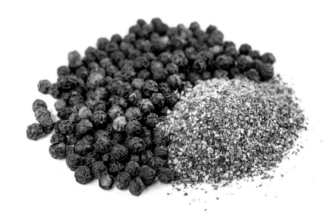

#7 – Cloves

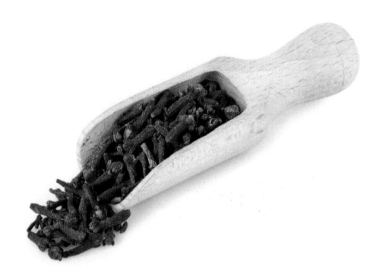

Numerous studies confirm the HIGH ANTIOXIDANT PROPERTIES of spices. A Spanish study went so far as to conclude that cloves are the "best" natural antioxidant [5]. As a metabolism enhancer, cloves are another spice that helps you lose weight. They assist the body in its ability to utilize food faster and more efficiently. This increased metabolism helps your body shed extra weight and avoid storing unneeded fat.

#8 – Cayenne

Hot peppers can be great for you! So, the next time you have the option to spice up some bland food, add some cayenne. Hot peppers like cayenne can be quite good for you. Medically, the body responds to a compound in cayenne pepper known as dihydrocapsiate which burns fat. BURN FAT... LOSE WEIGHT... SLIM DOWN... LOOK GOOD! Plus, this spice has healing potential - especially for colds. Spicy foods can help clear the mucus lining and keep your breathing passage clear.

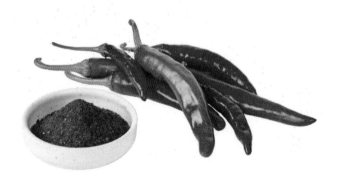

Rick Kaselj, MS, BSc, PK, CES
ExercisesForInjuries.com

Best Foods That Slim & Heal

#9 – Ginger

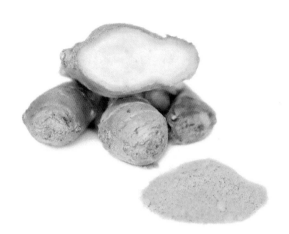

You can use this spice as the fresh root or in powdered form. Ginger has antioxidant and anti-inflammatory effects given its constituents, which include shogaol, gingerols and paradols that are also considered valuable cancer preventers [6]. Ginger provides a great tasting spice that can be used in a variety of dishes. In terms of weight loss, ginger tackles those frustrating food cravings. It controls appetite, which can contribute greatly to reducing calorie intake. Again, another great way to lose some weight.

#10 – Mustard

Spices burn calories! We've seen that already, and mustard is another one of these spices that can help you burn, burn, burn, burn those calories away. In essence, you get the nutrients you need by eating healthy foods, and spices like mustard help you utilize this food intake properly and more efficiently. You can consume mustard in the form of a paste, as is usually the case. However, there are also powdered forms of mustard, and mustard seeds.

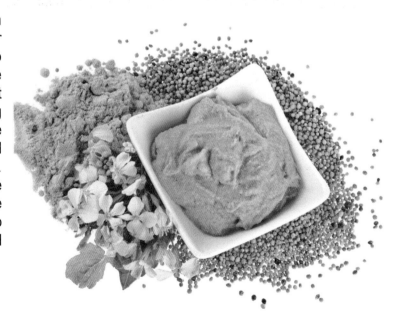

Rick Kaselj, MS, BSc, PK, CES
ExercisesForInjuries.com

45

#11 – Cardamom

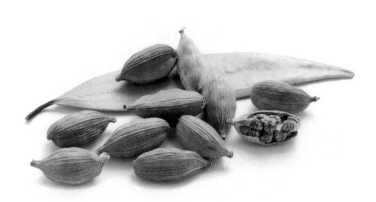

The cholesterol fighter, cardamom, fights the bad cholesterol that may have accumulated in the body. GREAT POINTS TO CARDAMOM for this! There is also the blood glucose lowering potential that cardamom offers in addition to managing insulin in the body. Reduced glucose in the body can contribute to a healthy weight.

#12 – Cumin

This spice has been associated with the digestive system and also in the transformation or conversion of food into energy. The digestive tract is incredibly IMPORTANT. If we have unhealthy digestive systems, our health is affected in many different ways. Essentially, the body could shut down due to nutrients not being absorbed properly. Skin conditions can occur and inflammation is another possibility. Therefore, consider cumin a life-saver, working to keep the digestive system happy!

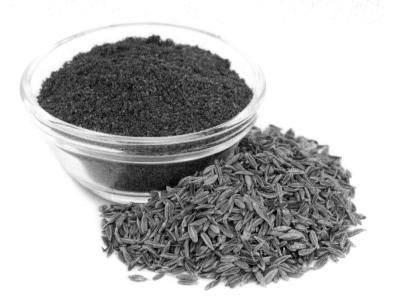

#13 – Coriander

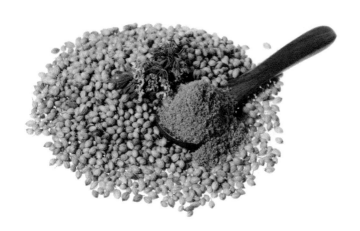

Coriander has nutritional and medicinal properties. This spice is full of nutrients, flavonoids and essential oils and can be used for stomach ailments, spasms, sedation, anti-diabetic activity, anticonvulsant, diuretic, anti-mutagenic activity and anti-microbial activities [7]. There are coriander seeds and leaves which provides you with options regarding how to incorporate this spice. QUITE NUTRIOUS and able to help you maintain good health and weight, coriander is worth giving a try!

#14 – Parsley

Then, there is parsley. Use parsley and tap into its ability to promote healthy conversion of food into energy. Parsley can be incorporated into meals in fresh leaf form or as dry flakes. There have been connections between parsley and appetite control. This is another area where research in ongoing. However, there is no denying that parsley has low calories. This makes it great as an ingredient in meals. Don't look at parsley the same way again! Instead, think about what parsley can do for you.

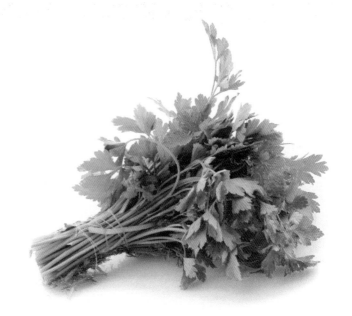

Spices can SPICE UP our lives ... literally ... and in ways that go beyond merely providing us with great tasting foods. You can use spices to maintain your weight. Spices can help you burn FAT! Spices can also enhance metabolism and support the conversion of fat into energy. They are wonderful for weight loss! In addition, THERE ARE MEDICINAL BENEFITS of spices. There is no reason not to include spices in your meals.

References

[1] The total antioxidant content of more than 3100 foods, beverages, spices, herbs and supplements used worldwide.: http://www.ncbi.nlm.nih.gov/pubmed/20096093

[2] Crocus sativus L. (saffron) for cancer chemoprevention: A mini review.: http://www.ncbi.nlm.nih.gov/pubmed/26151016

[3] Saffron (Crocus sativus) aqueous extract and its constituent crocinreduces stress-induced anorexia in mice.: http://www.ncbi.nlm.nih.gov/pubmed/21503997

[4] Assessment of antimycotoxigenic and antioxidant activity of star anise (*Illiciumverum*) *in vitro*: http://www.sciencedirect.com/science/article/pii/S1658077X14000368

[5] Cloves are 'best' natural antioxidant, Spanish study finds: http://www.sciencedaily.com/releases/2010/03/100316124231.htm

[6] Anti-Oxidative and Anti-Inflammatory Effects of Ginger in Health and Physical Activity: Review of Current Evidence: http://www.ncbi.nlm.nih.gov/pmc/articles/PMC3665023/

[7] Nutritional and medicinal aspects of coriander: http://www.academia.edu/8172447/Nutritional_and_medicinal_aspects_of_coriander_Coriandrum_sativum_L._A_review

Rick Kaselj, MS, BSc, PK, CES
ExercisesForInjuries.com

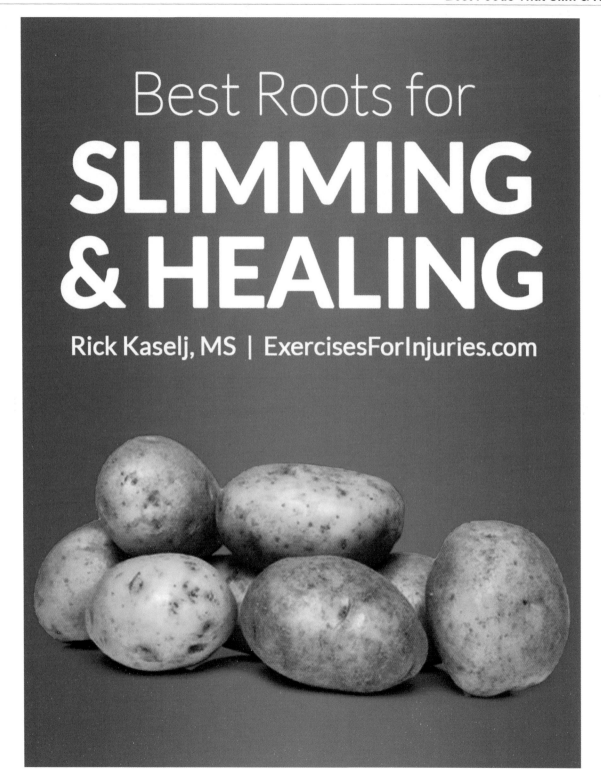

#1 – Beets

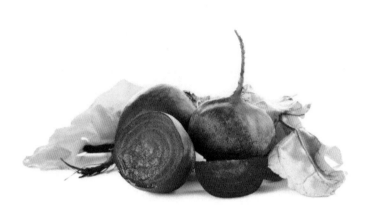

Bright and dark red in color, beets are a wonderful root containing lots of nutrients including vitamins C, B1, B2, B3, B6 and B9. Beets also contain protein, carbohydrates, calcium, phosphorus, fiber, iodine, iron, copper and other nutrients. There have been claims that beetroot improves athletic performance and can be used to treat heart failure patients [2]. With such a rich NUTRITIONAL profile, beets can be used in curing ailments such as anemia, as they rejuvenate the red blood cells and encourage normal cell functioning by supporting renewed supplies of oxygen.

#2 – Burdock Root

Another root that helps to detoxify the body is the burdock root. This root is great for weight loss because of its low-calorie count. With only 72 calories in a 100g portion of the root, you're able to gain some great nutrients and reduce unneeded pounds. CONTROL WEIGHT with a conscious addition of this root to your meals. You'll also reap benefits that include cholesterol and blood sugar control, blood pressure and heart

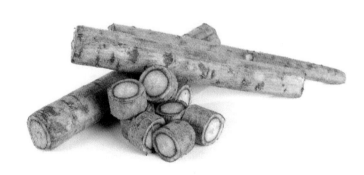

rate regulation, and improvements to skin conditions. Look and feel great with burdock root!

Rick Kaselj, MS, BSc, PK, CES
ExercisesForInjuries.com

#3 – Parsnips

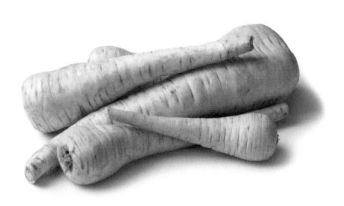

A good source of fiber, both soluble and insoluble, parsnips provide about 5mg of fiber in 100g portions. This fiber is great for the digestive system and also tackles constipation and cholesterol levels. Nutrients that can be found in parsnips include vitamin B9, potassium, vitamin C and manganese. Parsnips can be quite sweet and have been used as sugar substitutes.

#4 – Turnips

A great source of vitamin A, turnips can be used to provide healing to many conditions that respond to this particular vitamin. Turnips also contain vitamin E and have a significant amount of fiber. Some healing associated with turnips include ailments such as blood clots, heart disease and cancer. A GOOD source of health benefits while keeping your calorie count under control, turnips are quite good for you!

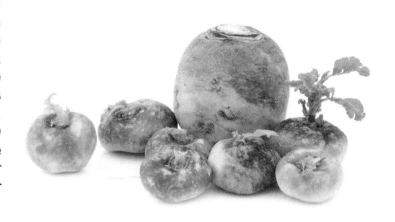

Rick Kaselj, MS, BSc, PK, CES
ExercisesForInjuries.com

#5 – Rutabagas

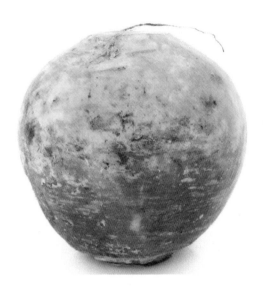

Quite the melodic name, rutabagas have Swedish origins; the word meaning "root". Loads of nutrients in this root provide a powerful healing mechanism for the body to draw from. In rutabagas, you'll find vitamins K, B1, B2, E, B3, B5 and B6. Rutabagas also contain copper, manganese, sodium, zinc, iron and calcium. WOW! All these nutrients in one root! Yes, rutabagas are quite the nutritional powerhouse.

#6 – Yacon Root

This root has Peruvian origins but can also be found in other parts of the world. The yacon root can now be found in countries in North America and the United Kingdom. One way that yacon root heals is through the presence of prebioticinulin. This root also contains fiber for the health of your digestive track and minerals such as magnesium. Use yacon root in salads or peel and slice it as a snack. You'll reap benefits that include weight loss and healing of your gut, increased bone health and gastrointestinal tract.

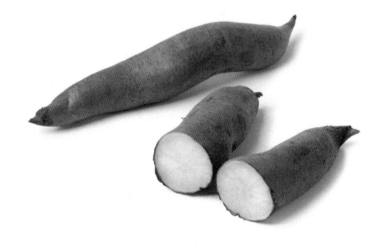

#7 – Chicory

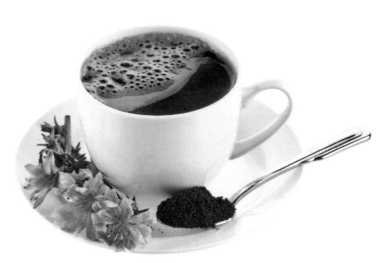

Known as a laxative, chicory targets the digestive system. In addition, chicory can aid the gallbladder and liver by helping to eliminate toxins. A unique quality about the chicory root is the ability to eat all parts of this plant. You can eat not only the roots, but also the leaves and buds. The plant is great for weight loss because it has insulin, helping to keep blood sugar levels in check. In terms of healing, chicory root uses its vitamins and minerals like vitamins C, A, B3, calcium, zinc and iron to fortify and provide restoration to the body.

#8 – Chinese Rhubarb Root

Where do we start with the nutritional and medicinal properties of the Chinese rhubarb root? It has anti-inflammatory, antibiotic and antibacterial properties which are core healing and defense mechanisms. It can help fight skin conditions such as acne, eczema, poison oak and much more! Studies show that rhubarb has some effect in treating the herpes simplex virus, which causes infections, cold sores and blisters [3]. It can also be used as a cleanser to take care of the

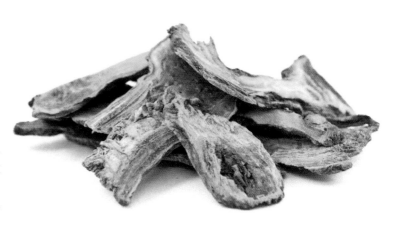

intestinal tract and the excretion of toxins from the body. Yes, it helps the liver too! There are many wonderful benefits of the Chinese rhubarb root!!

#9 – Horseradish

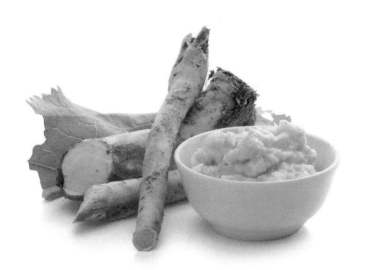

With just a small bite of horseradish you will feel the powerful punch this root provides. Horseradish may increase your appetite, though. So, make sure you are seeking the right foods if this occurs. Horseradish is low calorie, helping to contribute to weight loss. The root contains lots of nutrients that are good for healing your body, including copper, manganese, magnesium, sodium, potassium and many vitamins such as B2, B3, B5, B6 and B9. Research studies show that horseradish can be used in cancer therapy, bioremediation, biocatalysis and biosensor systems [4]. You can use horseradish to treat infections and inflammation too. Horseradish also contains vitamin C, which is another wonderful healing vitamin.

#10 – Daikon

Daikon is a root you may not have heard much about. However, it is certainly worth knowing. From Asian origins, daikon is a type of radish that can help remove build-up in the body from dairy sources, acting as a purifier or cleanser to help flush out the system. Daikon has powerful DIGESTIVE ENZYMES that help regulate the body and keep us functioning effectively. Daikon also has antioxidant properties [5]. With lots of nutrients and its low-fat

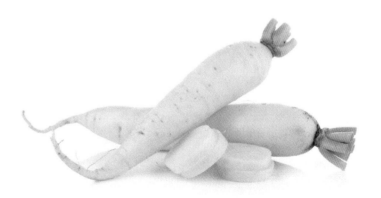

content, daikon is wonderful for weight loss. Its cleaning power also works to remove mucus and other substances that clog the respiratory system.

Rick Kaselj, MS, BSc, PK, CES
ExercisesForInjuries.com

#11 – Suma

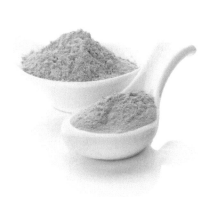

Used as an aphrodisiac, this root with its South American origins is known to relax and calm the body and mind. Although it can provide energy, it is also used as a sexual tonic. There have been links to the healing of ulcers when consuming this food. Suma is known to treat wounds, boost energy, treat cancer and many skin conditions [6]. It is quite popular among the tribes of the Amazon forest. Other uses of the suma root include the regulation of blood sugar levels and the stimulation of appetites.

#12 – Yams

These roots are not sweet potatoes! Popularly found in areas such as Asia or in Africa, yams usually come in different sizes, but are often long and tubular with varying lengths. What benefits do yams provide? Lots of minerals, including iron and manganese, vitamins B6, B9, C and fiber. In fact, yams are quite high in fiber, making them a good dietary choice. Yams also help fight bad cholesterol.

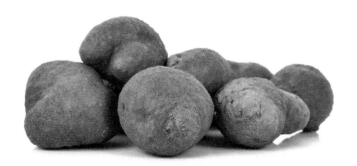

#13 – Yellow Dock Root

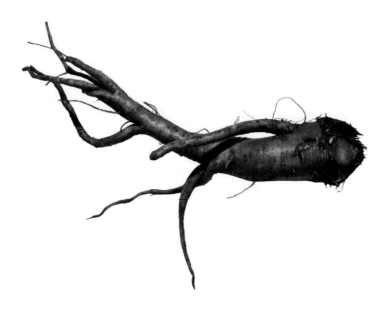

Yellow dock root is bitter to taste, but don't let this scare you away! Sometimes these bitter foods can do us a LOT OF GOOD! The yellow dock root can provide gallbladder and liver toning. It has also been reported that you can improve skin tone with this root. Yellow dock root is very high in iron. The root is low in fat, which is essential in keeping weight under control.

#14 – Ginger

Ginger is such a powerful root and wonderful to include in many dishes. Oh, the taste of ginger! And the delightful lemony aroma of the fresh cut root! Ginger has medicinal properties too. You can DETOX with ginger. You can LOSE WEIGHT with ginger. It also has anti-inflammatory properties that leave your skin looking healthier. A study showed that eating ginger can make you feel fuller, which aids in weight loss [7]. When you feel full, you eat less.

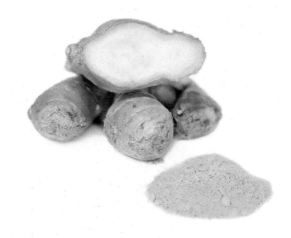

Rick Kaselj, MS, BSc, PK, CES
ExercisesForInjuries.com

It's no secret, roots can be MEDICINAL and have SLIMMING POTENTIAL too! Remember... in some parts of the world there is a core inclusion of roots as a main staple. You have the ability to make choices regarding the foods that you consume, and you can make better choices by adding these foods to your meals. ONE WAY to efficiently begin to eat more roots is to introduce them a little bit at a time... a few slices here and there, and before you know it, you'll be on your way to including more of these roots to YOUR benefit!

References

[1] Staple foods: What do people eat?: http://www.fao.org/docrep/u8480e/u8480e07.htm

[2] Beetroot beneficial for athletes, heart failure patients, research finds: http://www.sciencedaily.com/releases/2014/10/141023100938.htm

[3] University of Maryland Medical Center – Herpes simplex virus: http://umm.edu/health/medical-reference-guide/complementary-and-alternative-medicine-guide/condition/herpes-simplex-virus

[4] An updated view on horseradish peroxidases: recombinant production and biotechnological applications: http://www.ncbi.nlm.nih.gov/pmc/articles/PMC4322221/

[5] Antioxidant and Choleretic Properties of Raphanussativus L. Sprout (KaiwareDaikon) Extract: http://pubs.acs.org/doi/abs/10.1021/jf061838u

[6] Smart alternatives - Suma: http://www.altmd.com/Articles/Suma--Encyclopedia-of-Alternative-Medicine

[7] How to Lose Weight and Detox with Ginger: http://news.health.com/2012/12/31/how-to-lose-weight-and-detox-with-ginger/

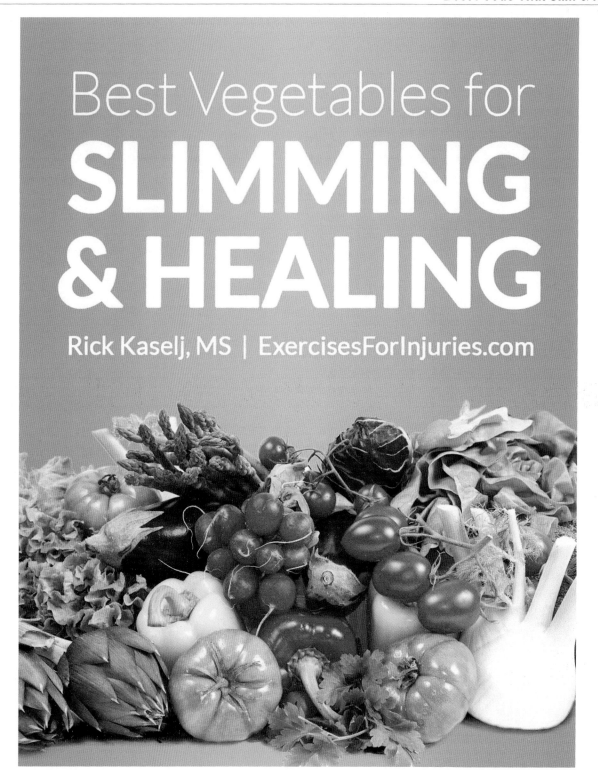

Best Vegetables for
SLIMMING
& HEALING

Rick Kaselj, MS | ExercisesForInjuries.com

#1 – Broccoli

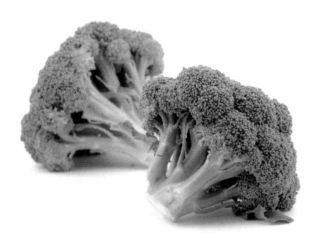

Do you like broccoli? Perhaps it's just not something that regularly makes it onto your lunch or dinner plate. Well... this is a great opportunity to re-think some of your choices. Broccoli is rich in vitamin C, which is essential for the prevention of infections and the healing of cuts. Broccoli also contains B vitamins for healthy red blood cells [2]. There is no fat in broccoli, which helps to enhance the opportunity for slimming while also providing healing for the body.

#2 – Fennel

Fennel has high potassium and calcium content, and contains flavonoids that tackle the free radicals in the body. These free radicals can end up making us feel sick and unhealthy. Fennel also has a unique flavor which makes it a great addition to foods such as salads and soups. Fennel is great for slimming and healing!

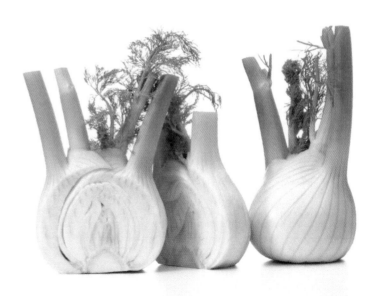

#3 – Kale

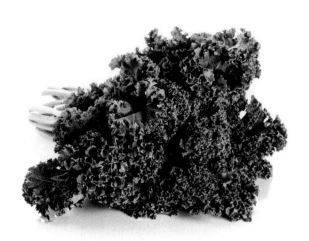

Kale has replaced lettuce on many dinner tables. It can help detoxify the body and also act as a blood cleanser. Quite wonderful! Next time you're looking for a HEALTHY SNACK, think about eating a kale salad or homemade kale chips instead. This is one way HEALTHY HABITS get formed.

#4 – Black Radish

A wonderful cruciferous plant, radishes are another vegetable worth including in your meals. There are different types of black radish, such as the Spanish black radish. Researchers studying Spanish black radish concluded that it has a positive influence on detoxification in the liver [3]. This is great news because the body functions more efficiently when it is cleansed of TOXINS! Toxins can frequently accumulate in the body and it is helpful to know that cruciferous vegetables can come to our RESCUE.

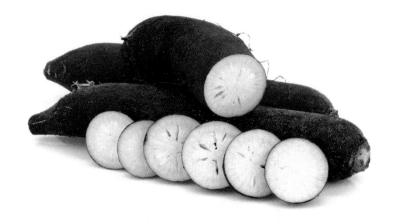

Rick Kaselj, MS, BSc, PK, CES
ExercisesForInjuries.com

#5 – Carrot

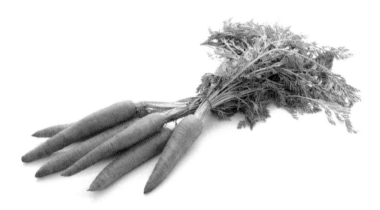

Apart from looking great with their bright orange color, carrots are good sources of fiber and can contribute to slimming goals as well! It can take LONGER to eat carrots than other snacks, especially in the raw or uncooked state. All this chewing keeps your mouth occupied and possibly less likely to overeat or take in too many calories! This is a great tip to remember when looking for a healthy snack!!

#6 – Cucumber

These vegetables have high water content. Cucumbers are quite succulent and great for juicing because of all that liquid content. In addition, cucumbers help keep the skin healthy and soothe away ailments that affect the muscles. Cucumber is a great addition to salads.

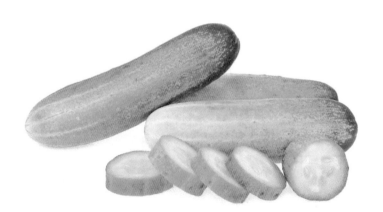

#7 – Celery

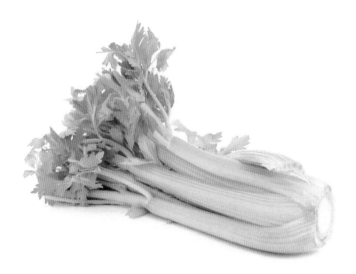

Another great vegetable for slimming is celery. Quite juicy too! Celery contains a significant amount of water, helping to hydrate the body. In addition, there are many medicinal benefits of celery, including the reduction of inflammation, regulating the alkaline balance of the body, stress relief and aiding in digestion. Celery has been used to treat arthritis, calm nerves and reduce inflammation. Animal studies also point to the reduction of blood pressure and cholesterol [4].

#8 – Cauliflower

How does cauliflower help you?... It can help with BLOOD PRESSURE REGULATION. There have also been connections between cauliflower and the reduced likelihood of heart disease and cancer. While most vegetables are quite low in calories, cauliflower is really low in calories and makes an excellent choice as a side dish when you are trying to manage or reduce your weight.

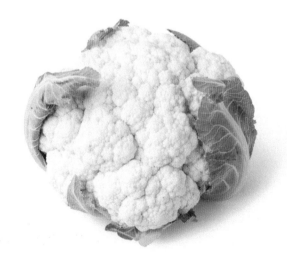

Rick Kaselj, MS, BSc, PK, CES
ExercisesForInjuries.com

#9 – Asparagus

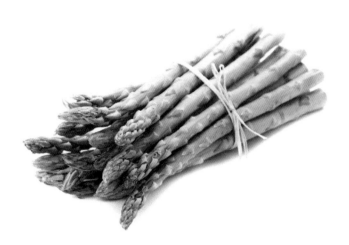

Asparagus can be somewhat stringy due to its HIGH FIBER content. High folate content makes this great for women who are pregnant. These vegetables also contain vitamin B6 and potassium. Replacing some of your bulky and less nutritious food options with asparagus could help you tremendously increase your intake of folate and other essential nutrients.

#10 – Lettuce

Leafy and full of goodness, research shows that lettuce is a source of antioxidant sphenolic extracts [5]. Also, research results show that lettuce seed oil has been used to gain improvements in patients suffering from insomnia [6]. There are many varieties of lettuce, so spruce up your salads with a variety of colors, textures and flavors. You are on a path to better health if you are consuming this vegetable.

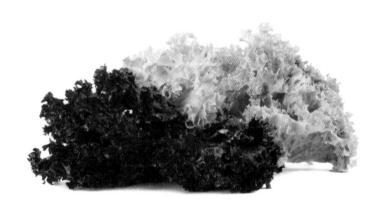

#11 – Leeks

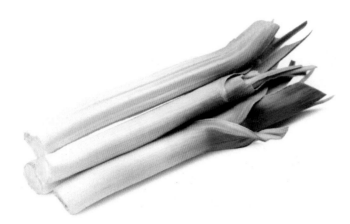

Leeks contain flavonoids and there are connections with this vegetable to reducing the risk of cancer. Leeks also contain vitamin B6, vitamin K and vitamin A. Leeks can reduce an amino acid in the blood known as homocysteine and also contain manganese [7].

#12 – Zucchini

A perfect summer vegetable, zucchini is a type of squash with tons of recipes and fun ways to consume this vegetable. Easy to obtain at farmers' markets and grocery stores, this is a healthy food with lots of flavor. Zucchinis are also referred to as courgettes. Grill or roast zucchinis for lunch or dinner. Zucchini contains very little calories and are a good source of nutrients. A 100g of zucchini contains ONLY 17 calories [8].

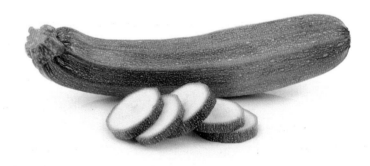

Rick Kaselj, MS, BSc, PK, CES
ExercisesForInjuries.com

#13 – Cabbage

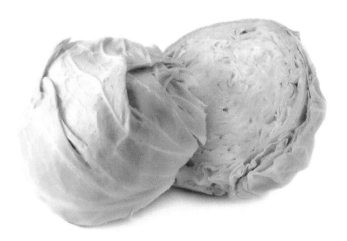

A low-calorie vegetable that you can count on, cabbage can be eaten in soups, salads, rolls and much more. Cabbage has been linked to the destruction of cancer cells when combined with traditional chemotherapy. It contains vital nutrients, anti-inflammatory compounds and antioxidants [9]. Its low-calorie count makes it great for weight loss, while its medicinal properties provide healing.

#14 – Endive

There are lots of species of the endive vegetable. Part of the chicory family, it has also been referred to as escarole. Like other vegetables, endive has low calories and provides LOTS of NUTRITIONAL VALUE. Endive's unique nutty flavor can make salads more flavorful. Some of the nutrients in endive include vitamins K, A, C, E, thiamin, folates and niacin. Research studies point to the use of endive for glucose and cholesterol reduction [10]. Other research has also shown that some types of anemia can be cured with endive [11].

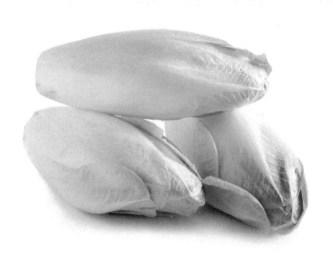

#15 – Spinach

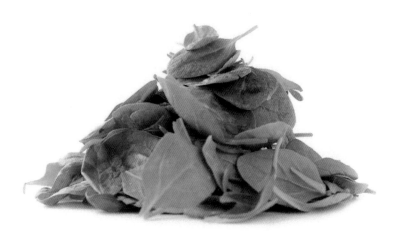

Spinach has been linked to strength in movies and has other pop culture connections. Indeed, spinach is a healthy option. In terms of slimming and losing weight, spinach can be a good vegetable to latch onto. If you are interested in losing some weight, throw a handful of spinach on your salads or try sautéing a bit of spinach in a pan to use as a side to your meals.

HOW WONDERFUL! You can CUT the FAT simply by eating vegetables. Sometimes, we don't include enough veggies in our meals because we don't know how. Don't worry - you are not alone! Simply begin by thinking about creative ways you can incorporate veggies into your dishes, bit by bit. Adding a little fruit to your veggies can help to make it easier and more FUN to consume!

References

[1] Healthy Kids – Eat More Fruit and Veggies: https://www.healthykids.nsw.gov.au/home/fact-sheets/eat-more-fruit-and-vegies.aspx

[2] Colour Your Choices with Vegetables and Fruit: http://www.dietitians.ca/Your-Health/Nutrition-A-Z/Canada-s-Food-Guide/Colour-your-choices-with-Vegetables-and-Fruit.aspx

[3] Efficacy of Spanish black radish on the induction of phase I and phase II enzymes in healthy male subjects: http://www.ncbi.nlm.nih.gov/pubmed/25490898

[4] University of Maryland Medical Center - Celery Seed: http://umm.edu/health/medical/altmed/herb/celery-seed

[5] Lettuce and chicory byproducts as a source of antioxidant phenolic extracts: http://www.ncbi.nlm.nih.gov/pubmed/15291483

[6] Pilot study of the efficacy and safety of lettuce seed oil in patients with sleep disorders: http://www.ncbi.nlm.nih.gov/pubmed/21731897

[7] Why leeks are good for you: http://www.theguardian.com/lifeandstyle/2014/jan/27/why-leeks-are-good-for-you

[8] Zucchini nutrition facts: http://www.nutrition-and-you.com/zucchini.html

[9] Cabbage proven to drastically risk reduce of cancer, contains anti-inflammatory compounds: http://www.naturalnews.com/049913_cabbage_benefits_cancer_prevention_natural_healing.html

[10] Endive nutrition facts and health benefits: http://www.nutrition-and-you.com/endive.html

[11] Megalocytic Deficiency Anaemia Cured By Small Amounts of Fresh Endive: http://www.ncbi.nlm.nih.gov/pmc/articles/PMC1988515/pdf/archdisch01414-0003.pdf

Rick Kaselj, MS, BSc, PK, CES
ExercisesForInjuries.com

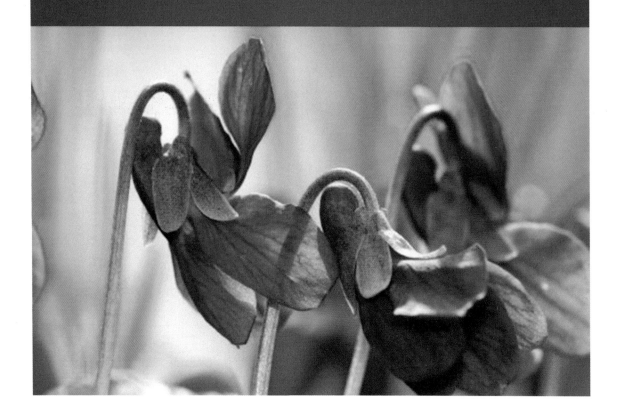

Best Flowers for
SLIMMING
& HEALING

Rick Kaselj, MS | ExercisesForInjuries.com

Best Flowers for Slimming and Healing

If I told you that flowers could be used for SLIMMING AND HEALING, would you believe me? Probably not, especially if you have only thought of flowers as something pretty to look at or something with a great fragrance to sniff and smell. However, flowers are SO MUCH MORE than looks and smells. You can use flowers for healing the body and for managing your weight. The U.S. National Library of Medicine has approximately 75 to 100 kinds of flowers and herbs in its garden, and these plants have a continually relevant and rich history of medicinal use [1]. Flowers and herbs really can help heal the body and help you get rid of those extra pounds!

But how? This answer is quite simple, really... flowers are natural sources of many powerful nutrients that work hard on the body to bring about healing, while burning calories too. There are flowers that help with weight loss. In addition, there are flowers that can heal; all sorts or types of healing including healing JOINT PAIN, GUT DAMAGE and helping with MUSCLE PAIN. Do you suffer from any of these ailments or perhaps you know someone who has complained of these conditions? If yes, this information is just what you need.

What if there was a way to rid yourself of such pain and damage to the body, and DO SO NATURALLY TOO! Yes, flowers are all natural... just what the body needs... no extra and unneeded processing of added compounds which could be difficult for the body to use or eliminate. No, you get a better deal with FLOWERS! So, tap into their healing and slimming power today!

Let's take a closer look at some of these powerful flowers, which can also be classified as herbs. Yes, these herbs are quite POWERFUL! This cannot be over-emphasized! Here is a list of flowers (powerful herbs) that can help get you on the path of slimming and healing...

Rick Kaselj, MS, BSc, PK, CES
ExercisesForInjuries.com

#1 - Foxglove

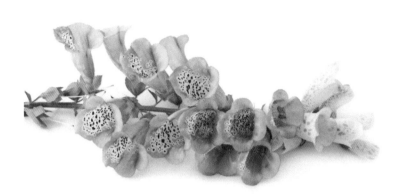

Herbs and flowers are quite powerful and can provide healing and weight management opportunities. However, care should be taken when using flowers for healing and slimming, as the excessive consumption of some of these flowers could be quite detrimental to the body. Foxglove is one of those flowers that need to be consumed in moderate amounts. There is the potential for foxglove poisoning [2], so use caution and stay informed.

This plant is great for healing colds and coughs. Foxglove flower is quite the cold infection buddy! You can also use foxglove flowers to treat swellings and puffiness that is associated with ailments like edema.

#2 - Lilac

Healing is part of what lilac does! Great for burns and wounds, lilac can be used for fevers too. Easily steep the petals of this flower in hot water to create a potent tonic that can be used to reduce fevers. The scent of lilac has a soothing effect. Its fragrance can help calm people or cause a person to prepare for rest.

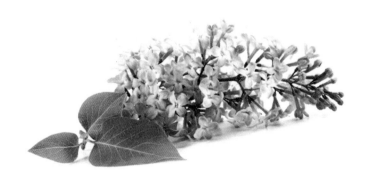

#3 - Butterfly Weed

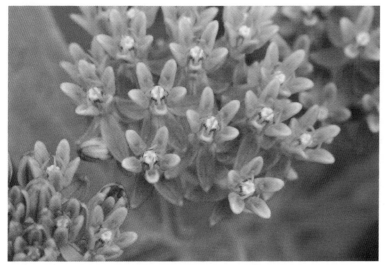

Don't let the "weed" included in the name of this flower fool you regarding its usefulness. On the contrary, butterfly weed is useful in a variety of treatments, including the treatment of swelling, skin issues, lung ailments and healing wounds. Why is it named "butterfly weed"? Good question! This plant has brightly colored flowers that attract butterflies to it.

#4 - California Poppy

If you are having problems sleeping, you could use California poppy to treat insomnia and get a good night's rest. Yes, calm the body with an infused blend of California poppy. Research studies show that the California poppy can also be used to treat pain [3]. There are connections between California poppy and fighting off fatigue. People with depression can also get some relief with the use of California poppy.

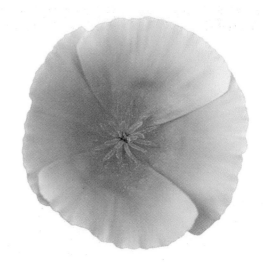

Rick Kaselj, MS, BSc, PK, CES
ExercisesForInjuries.com

#5 - Dandelion

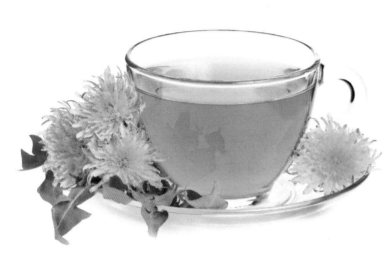

Another powerful flower that takes aim at blood ailments is dandelion. Dandelion is used for cleansing the blood and when we consider how important the blood is, we can see how beneficial this flower is. People who are anaemic could find this quite beneficial. Dandelion tonics are used to achieve a sense of well-being and consuming the herb or flower has no adverse effect on your weight.

#6 - Rosy Periwinkle

This flower has a delightful name as well as wonderful healing properties. The rosy periwinkle has been used to treat conditions such as high blood pressure. There have also been associations between the use of rosy periwinkle and the treatment of cancer and leukemia. There can be some toxicity associated with the rosy periwinkle plant, even though medicinal effects have been established [4]. Hence, caution is also advised.

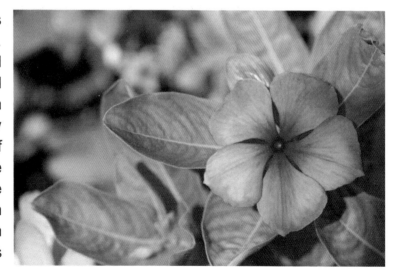

Rick Kaselj, MS, BSc, PK, CES
ExercisesForInjuries.com

#7 - Peony

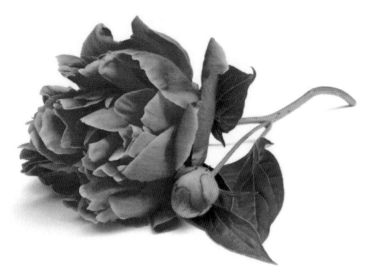

This is another flower that is great as a tonic. Use peony to help relax muscles and ease tension. If you experience cramps for any variety of reasons, including menstrual discomfort, you'll be glad to have a drink of peony tonic nearby.

#8 - Sunflower

Another flower that is good for those menstrual or other types of cramping is the sunflower. Extensive research on the sunflower shows that this plant has a positive effect on the skin [5]. Usually, a tonic made with sunflower is consumed to help treat pains, sore throats, cramps and ulcers. Applications from the sunflower plant also include sunflower seeds and sunflower oil.

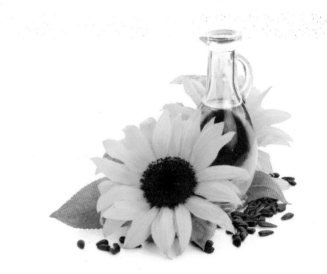

Rick Kaselj, MS, BSc, PK, CES
ExercisesForInjuries.com

#9 - May Apple

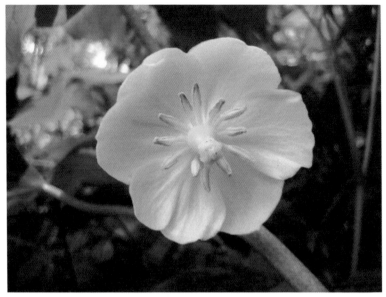

A powerful herb and flower, may apple can sometimes be too powerful, so DO BEWARE. Care should be taken when using this flower, as it can also be toxic to the body. There is a need to balance its medicinal properties with its limitations. It does have laxative properties, but you do need the help of a professionally trained specialist with knowledge of herbs and plants to help you determine adequate dosage levels when consuming may apple.

#10 - Hyssop

If you gargle a tonic made with hyssop flowers, you can feel your sore throat ease. Quite the effective treatment for chest ailments too, including congestion and bronchitis. Good for arthritis, you can use hyssop to get rid of the pain in the joints as it aids with blood circulation in the body.

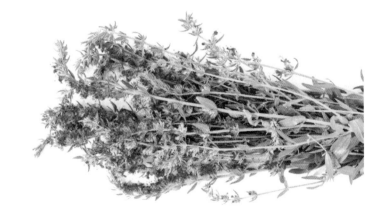

#11 - Gardenia

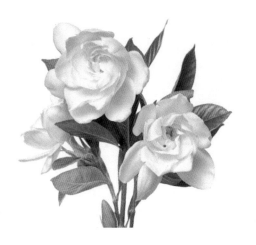

Gardenias are a popular flower and have deep usage in China for blood related disorders or cleansing. Other uses of gardenias include battling depression, as this flower appears to provide a 'lifting' feeling and in turn releases the body from the depressive state. So, yes... gardenia flowers operate on many levels, including mentally helping the body heal.

#12 - Carnations

A great tea and wonderful to consume (even without any noticeable ailment), carnation tea provides a calming effect. Now, who doesn't need that? There are also treatment possibilities associated with the reduction of swelling and helping the skin reduce puffiness. If you feel bloating, this tea not only calms your mind but also heals your body.

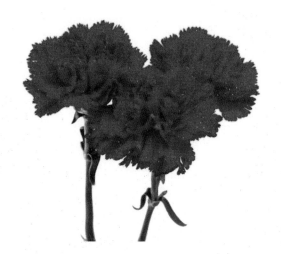

Rick Kaselj, MS, BSc, PK, CES
ExercisesForInjuries.com

#13 - Lotus

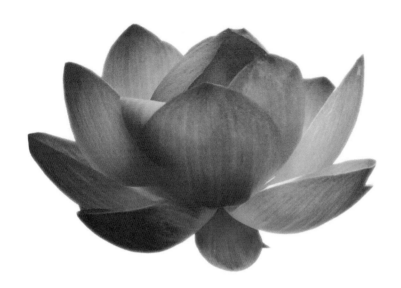

One application of the lotus flower is in treating tummy upsets including diarrhea, and chronic illnesses like bronchitis. You could also use lotus syrup to treat diseases like cholera. However, it is more popularly associated with respiratory tract infections and ailments like coughs. You can also use lotus to help the kidneys, spleen and heart [6]. Quite a powerful plant!!

#14 - Roses

Roses are beautiful, right? However, did you know that roses are also a good source of vitamin C? And what does vitamin C do for your body? HEALING! There are also connections between roses and blood circulation. Rose petals have been used in drinks or infused in water, and can also be a treatment for depression. Have you heard about rose tea? Well, if you have, now you know why this tea can be beneficial to you.

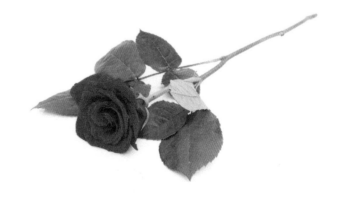

I bet you never thought flowers could be so powerful, right? Flowers are perfect for healing and slimming too. What you need to remember about these flowers is that they are herbs too. Hence, we are talking about LOW, LOW CALORIES! A perfect combination – slimming and healing, simply by using flowers!

References

[1] U.S. National Library of Medicine – List of Herbs: http://www.nlm.nih.gov/about/herbgarden/list.html

[2] MedlinePlus – Foxglove poisoning: https://www.nlm.nih.gov/medlineplus/ency/article/002878.htm

[3] California poppy for pain – does it really work?: http://www.emaxhealth.com/8782/california-poppy-pain-does-it-really-work

[4] Rosy periwinkle – A life saving plant: http://www.foxnews.com/health/2013/07/31/rosy-periwinkle-life-saving-plant/

[5] Effect of olive and sunflower seed oil on the adult skin barrier: implications for neonatal skin care: http://www.ncbi.nlm.nih.gov/pubmed/22995032

[6] Medicinal uses of lotus seed and other lotus plant parts: http://www.mdidea.com/products/proper/proper0666705.html

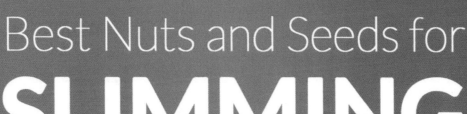

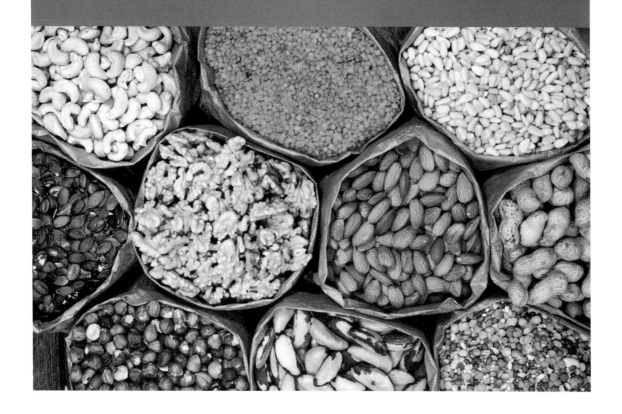

Best Nuts and Seeds for Slimming and Healing

There are many different kinds of nuts and seeds. For those who are able to consume these foods, you are tapping into a world of nourishment, great benefits related to healing of the body, and weight management too! Nuts and seeds are rich sources of unsaturated fats and can help reduce inflammation, cardiovascular disease and the risk of diabetes [1].

Why are nuts and seeds so good for you? Well... the nutritional profiles of these foods are LOADED with really good stuff! Vitamins and minerals that you need for healing can easily be found in nuts and seeds. The following nuts and seeds are some of the best available for slimming and healing.

#1 - Chia

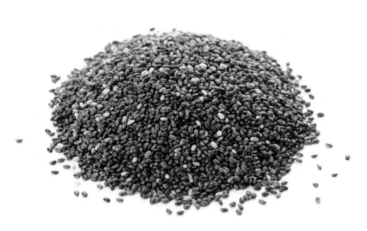

The Journal of Biomedicine and Biotechnology describes a research study depicting the promising future of chia. Chia has numerous health benefits, including the maintenance of healthy serum lipid levels [2]. Indeed, some would call chia ONE OF THE HEALTHIEST foods available, with nutrients that can do a world of good for both your body and your mind. Chia has lots of antioxidants for healing of the body. In addition, you'll get calcium, protein and fiber. Really... all this NUTRITION in little, tiny chia seeds!

Rick Kaselj, MS, BSc, PK, CES
ExercisesForInjuries.com

#2 - Flaxseeds

Flaxseeds are able to contribute effectively to daily dietary fiber requirements. 100g of flaxseed can provide 108% of the required daily value. That's over 100% from only 100 grams! Hence, this seed tackles issues associated with low fiber in the diet. There is also research regarding flaxseeds that show medicinal benefits. As a result of its large omega-3 fatty acid component, flaxseeds have significant cardiovascular effects, including cholesterol-lowering actions [3].

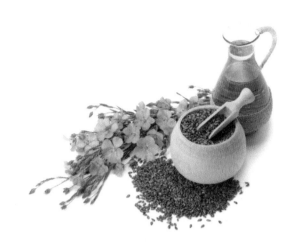

#3 - Sesame Seeds

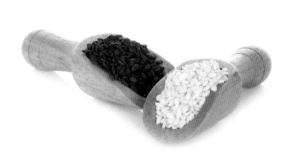

Typically found in regions of Africa and India, sesame seeds are great for sprinkling on, or adding to many dishes and baked goods. However, sesame seeds are much more valuable than how they look. Sesame seeds are a low glycemic food and a great source of antioxidants as well. They are also a good source of dietary fiber. Sesame seeds are quite appealing to many people – offering a nutty and flavourful experience! They are great for your health and waistline too.

#4 - Chestnuts

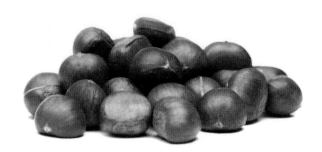

Any chestnuts roasting? Well, it may not be the season for it (or perhaps it is). Nevertheless, grab some chestnuts. In addition to the usual vitamins that nuts have, such as B1, B2 and B6, chestnuts contain vitamins C and K that are great for the body. You also get a reasonable amount of protein from just a few roasted chestnuts. With 2.7 grams of protein and just 200 calories in 10 to 12 pieces, chestnuts are great for snacking and weight management.

#5 - Almonds

Great as a snack or tossed into salads, almonds are a great nut to have handy. Roughly 23 nuts can provide 6 grams of protein and at least 3 grams of fiber. You'll also get a lot of vitamins from this nutty delight, including vitamin B1 (thiamine), vitamin B2 (riboflavin), vitamin B6, folate, niacin and vitamin E. Don't forget the minerals too, including zinc, copper, manganese, calcium, phosphorous, iron,

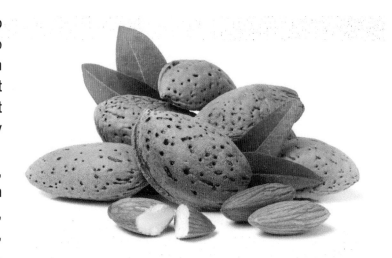

magnesium and potassium. Really... how can you go wrong in terms of healing with almonds? They have vitamins, minerals, protein and fiber! ALL THESE NUTIRENTS help you stay fit and healthy.

Rick Kaselj, MS, BSc, PK, CES
ExercisesForInjuries.com

#6 - Walnuts

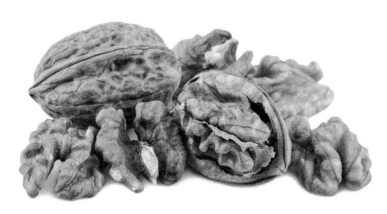

This is another powerful nut with lots of health benefits including helping your heart remain healthy, a cancer fighter, managing weight, reproductive health, treating or managing diabetes, and contributing to brain health. Walnuts contain significant amounts of antioxidants and help with overall health [4]. They also contain elements that protect the neurological system, including folate, antioxidants, omega-3 fatty acids and melatonin. Let's not forget that they contain vitamin E too.

#7 - Hemp Seeds

These may also be referred to as hemp hearts. When you think of hemp seeds, think LOADS of PROTEIN! These seeds are also packed with a lot of nutrients. In addition, you can use hemp seeds in a variety of ways. You can choose to consume these seeds raw, in hemp milk, or in baked goods. There's a lot of nutritious content; protein, omega-3 fatty acids... plus lots and lots of usage and consumption options.

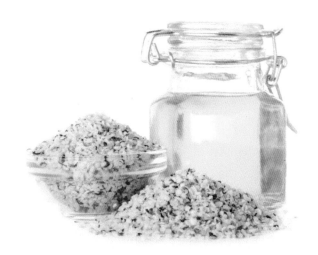

Rick Kaselj, MS, BSc, PK, CES
ExercisesForInjuries.com

#8 - Pecans

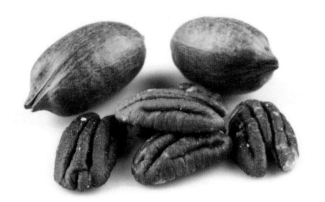

Related to hickory, pecans have origins that include areas of North America. Although high in fat, pecans are still said to have a really good nutrition profile and generally help to promote good health. Pecans contain antioxidants that are great for HEALING. You'll also get vitamins, minerals and fiber when you eat pecans. 100 grams of pecans can provide 9 grams of protein. Not bad at all! Other nutrients found in pecans include magnesium, iron, vitamin C, calcium, vitamin B6 and vitamin A.

#9 - Pistachios

Researchers from Penn State University discuss study results showing that pistachios have multiple health benefits, including heart-healthy connections, lower cholesterol levels and high levels of antioxidants [5]. Yes, there is the fat content to consider (a one ounce serving of pistachios will provide 160 calories), but you are also getting a LOT of nutrition. It is definitely worth it for your HEART! You get vitamins, minerals, fiber and protein in a serving of pistachios.

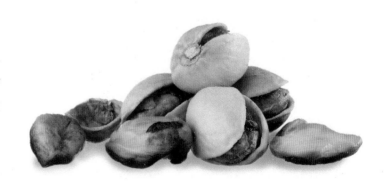

Rick Kaselj, MS, BSc, PK, CES
ExercisesForInjuries.com

#10 – Quinoa

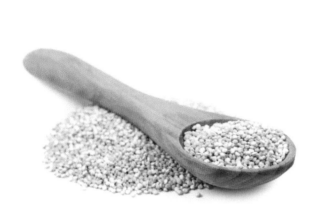

Known as one of the ancient grains, quinoa is great to have in your cupboard! This ancient grain originated from regions around Columbia, Peru and Bolivia. There have also been origins of the grain linked to Ecuador. No matter where this wonderful grain originated, the great news is that it's here! A low-calorie food, quinoa has edible seeds that can be prepared in a variety of ways. It is also rich in protein and fiber. A news article in the Telegraph news outlet highlighted a professor from Harvard University commenting on the life-saving properties of quinoa, and described how people who ate 34 grams of whole grains per day lowered their risk of dying prematurely by 17% [6]. Quinoa is a dual combination of healing and has the potential of keeping you full and slim. It's quite the versatile food!

Nuts and seeds; a food category that YOU SHOULD consider including in your diet if you are not already doing so. Let's face it, we need the nutrients that nuts and seeds provide. Dietary guidelines encourage individuals to consume foods that are nutrient-dense, such as nuts and seeds. There have been outcomes related to such consumption that include improved cardiovascular health [7]. It's right there... protein and antioxidants for your healing and strength, with vitamins and minerals to further fortify your body and keep you in the best shape. Let's not forget the fiber! Oh, the fiber! You need this to help keep your body functioning well. In essence, you can lose weight despite these nuts and seeds containing some fat. These are the GOOD FATS, and other nutrients in nuts and seeds help to heal ailments like joint pain and gut damage, while also helping you deal with muscle pain. What are you waiting for? Tap into the wonderfully nutritious world of nuts and seeds.

References

[1] Nut and seed consumption and inflammatory markers in the multi-ethnic study of atherosclerosis: http://www.ncbi.nlm.nih.gov/pubmed/16357111

[2] The Promising Future of Chia - NCBI: http://www.ncbi.nlm.nih.gov/pmc/articles/PMC3518271/

[3] The cardiovascular effects of flaxseed and its omega-3 fatty acid, alpha-linolenic acid: http://www.ncbi.nlm.nih.gov/pmc/articles/PMC2989356/

[4] Antioxidant activity comparison of walnuts and fatty fish: http://www.ncbi.nlm.nih.gov/pubmed/23130505

[5] Pistachios offer multiple health benefits: http://news.psu.edu/story/167129/2010/05/20/research/pistachios-offer-multiple-health-benefits

[6] Daily bowl of quinoa could save your life says Harvard University: http://www.telegraph.co.uk/news/science/science-news/11490006/Daily-bowl-of-quinoa-could-save-your-life-says-Harvard-University.html

[7] Centers for Disease Control and Prevention – Nut Consumption Among U.S. Adults 2009-2010: http://www.cdc.gov/nchs/data/databriefs/db176.htm

Rick Kaselj, MS, BSc, PK, CES
ExercisesForInjuries.com

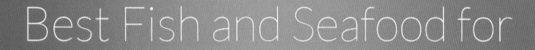

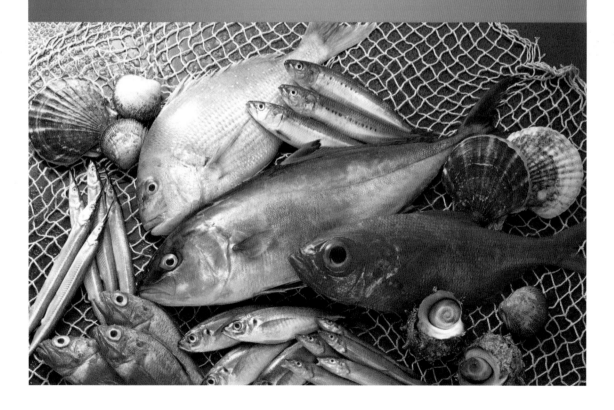

Best Fish & Seafood for Slimming and Healing

Fish and seafood can be quite GOOD for the body. While there is information available that encourages people to eat more seafood, there are also cautionary remarks regarding eating certain types of fish. Fish and seafood are the richest source of fatty acids, known as omega-3 fatty acids. These fatty acids can help in the treatment and prevention of diseases such as cancer, diabetes, mental disorders, heart disease, inflammation, diabetes, digestive disorders, autoimmune disease and high blood pressure [1]. Why is fish so POWERFUL as a category of food to eat? Well... as we just read, fish contains fish oils which are basically omega-3 fatty acids. These fish oils are an anti-inflammatory substance, and can also act as alternative anti-inflammatory and non-steroidal drugs capable of tackling pain [2].

Why is this so important? Well, our bodies do not make omega-3 fatty acids and these acids are essential to the body. So, how do we get these nutrients into our bodies? THROUGH FISH AND SEAFOOD!! The goal is to get to the best fish and seafood out there... those that can keep you trim and assist with healing! With so many types of fish out there, how do we manage to find the best ones to eat? Many fish look and taste similar, especially when cooked in a certain way.

No worries! We will guide you, and once you latch on to the right type of fish, it can be great for you and your waistline. Packed with nutrients yet still low calorie, fish is exactly what you want to keep slim and trim. So, what are these best seafood and fish to include in your meals? Let's take a look!

Rick Kaselj, MS, BSc, PK, CES
ExercisesForInjuries.com

#1 - Trout

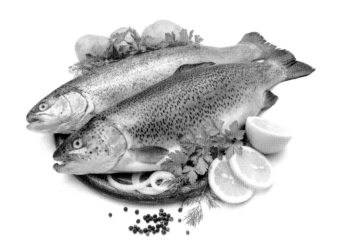

Trout is described as an excellent source of omega-3 fatty acids. It provides the World Health Organization's recommended daily serving of 300 to 500 mg of both docosahexanoic acid (DHA) and eicosapentanoic acid (EPA) [3]. A really great source of protein, did you know that 3 ounces of trout contains 21 grams of protein? All this powerful protein for your body by merely eating some trout! I bet you'll never look at trout the same way again! Protein consumption can help you build muscle mass, look lean and keep fit.

#2 - Wild Salmon

Although salmon contains a high fat content, these are fats the that can be good for you. When it comes to the consumption of fat that can lead to WEIGHT LOSS, salmon is great! In addition, eating salmon has been linked to the REDUCTION OF INFLAMMATION in the body. Wild salmon can be much leaner than salmon that comes from fish farms, as farmed fish are fed a certain type of food that can adversely "FATTEN" them up. It's easy to see why wild salmon can be a much healthier choice!

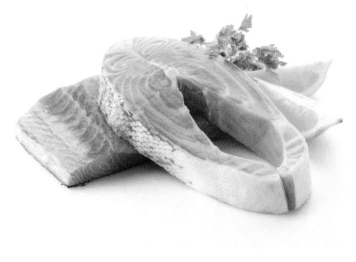

Rick Kaselj, MS, BSc, PK, CES
ExercisesForInjuries.com

#3 - Oysters

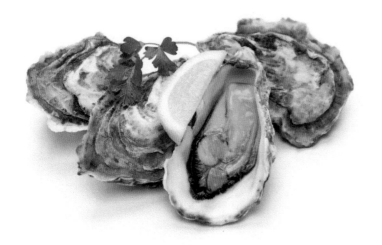

Oysters have low calorie content, which makes them a great addition to meals. Three oysters equate to about 22 calories! Easily reduce your calorie count by simply adding oysters to a dish or making them the main component of your meal. Appetite regulation is associated with oysters. Thus, you may be able to control those undesirable food cravings that cause you to overeat.

#4 - Mackerel

"Oily fish" like mackerel are considered some of the healthiest types of fish to consume. With fish like mackerel, you'll be able to lower the risk of heart disease that can often lead to premature death [4]. Apart from being a source of valuable fatty acids, fish like mackerel also provide nutrients, vitamins and minerals. Research studies show that mackerel as part of a person's diet can help to lower

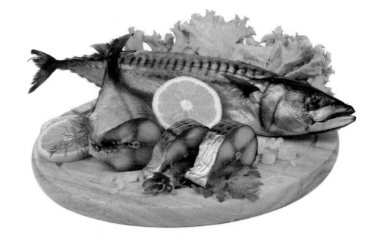

blood pressure. Even a low-dose regimen can effectively lower blood pressure that is mildly elevated [5].

#5 - Halibut

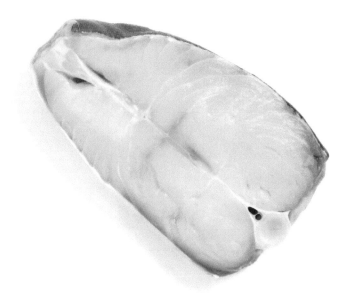

Have you ever had a fish meal and felt really full afterwards? Yes, fish can be very filling. Halibut can provide you with significant amounts of fiber. Yes, fiber! Who would have known that fish could be a great source of fiber?

#6 - Scallops

Ahh... scallops. It can be quite challenging to find dishes containing scallops that are not loaded with calories. However, it is generally the way that scallops are prepared and served that accounts for this increased calorie count. Especially in restaurants, when prepared by professional chefs, scallops can be subject to creamy delights and mouth watering creations that are not conducive to any tangible weight loss plan. That being said, scallops

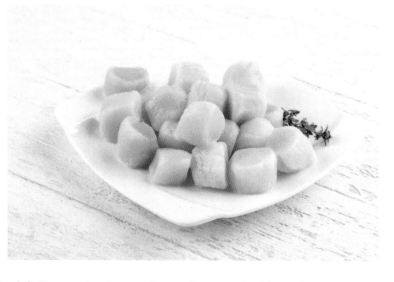

by themselves, without too much added fatty content, can be quite good at keeping you trim and fit. In terms of helping the body to heal, scallops tackle blood cholesterol with the aim of lowering it.

Rick Kaselj, MS, BSc, PK, CES
ExercisesForInjuries.com

#7 - Pacific Cod

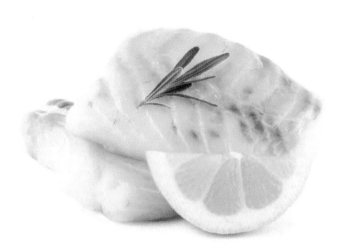

Another great fish for weight loss, pacific cod is one type of fish you should definitely be eating. It is great for weight loss in terms of its low-calorie count. Comparatively, foods with similar calorie counts may not provide the same sort of weight loss potential that pacific cod does!

#8 - Tuna

Easily affordable in most cases, tuna is one fish that people are able to find and typically buy without breaking the bank. In addition, tuna is GOOD for you. Tuna is known as a great source of docosahexaenoic acid (DHA). DHA is able to tone the gut and abdomen, keeping you looking and feeling slim and healthy. There have been high mercury levels linked to large tuna fish. However, smaller tuna have been known to have lower levels of mercury.

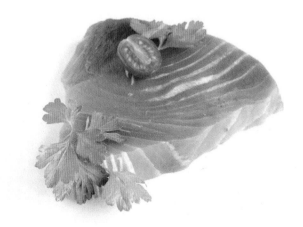

Rick Kaselj, MS, BSc, PK, CES
ExercisesForInjuries.com

#9 - Herring

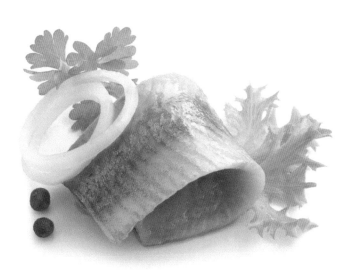

Eating the right kinds of fish is important. Herring is another fish that contains high amounts of omega-3 fatty acids. These fatty acids can reduce triglycerides or bad fats, lower blood pressure, decrease the likelihood of stroke, minimize heart failure risk, increase learning ability and reduce irregular heartbeats [6].

#10 - Sardines

These fish may be tiny, but can have a big impact on overall health and maintaining a healthy weight. Sardines are available fresh or in cans, and effectively retain their powerful source of omega-3 fatty acids. Sardines can come in small cans, making it convenient to transport or carry along with you. This type of fish is also quite affordable.

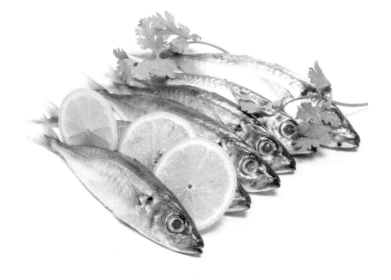

Fish and seafood can provide anti-inflammatory properties that help with healing and recovery. This is such an essential component of treatment for various ailments that can leave the body's cells, muscles, ligaments and tissues in need of repair. Eating fish that is high in omega-3 fatty acids can be really good for you. While oysters, tuna, halibut and scallops have moderate levels of omega-3 fatty acids, fish like trout, mackerel and wild salmon contain high omega-3 fatty acids. Eat fish and stay healthy and slim.

References

[1] University of Michigan –Integrative Medicine – Healing Foods Pyramid: http://www.med.umich.edu/umim/food-pyramid/fish.html

[2] Omega-3 fatty acids (fish oil) as an anti-inflammatory: an alternative to nonsteroidal anti-inflammatory drugs for discogenic pain.: http://www.ncbi.nlm.nih.gov/pubmed/16531187

[3] Is Trout Good for You?: http://healthyeating.sfgate.com/trout-good-you-2923.html

[4] University of Maryland Medical Center – Heart-Healthy Diet: http://umm.edu/health/medical/reports/articles/hearthealthy-diet

[5] Blood pressure-lowering effect of mackerel diet: http://www.ncbi.nlm.nih.gov/pubmed/2189040

[6] Omega-3 in fish: How eating fish helps your heart: http://www.mayoclinic.org/diseases-conditions/heart-disease/in-depth/omega-3/art-20045614

About Rick Kaselj

Rick Kaselj, M.S. (Exercise Science), B.Sc. (Kinesiology), PK, CPT, CEP, CES

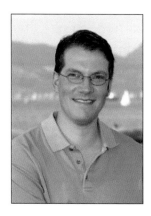

Hi, I'm Rick Kaselj. **I create exercise programs that help people heal injuries and eliminate pain, so they can go back to living a full, active, healthy life.**

I've always been a fitness and exercise enthusiast, so starting in 1994, I decided to make this my career. I started as a personal trainer, exercise therapist and kinesiologist, but quickly discovered that many of the traditional exercise and treatment programs available weren't producing the results I wanted for my clients.

I took it upon myself to get the right knowledge, scour the medical research, and do hands-on testing, so I could ACTUALLY help my clients get better.

With the advent of the Internet, I saw a terrific opportunity to offer expand my reach and deliver my programs to many more people, so they too could finally get relief from pain, heal their injuries, and get back to the lives they enjoy.

I USE RESEARCH, STUDY, AND HANDS-ON TESTING TO FIND WHAT <u>REALLY</u> <u>WORKS</u> TO HEAL INJURIES AND ELIMINATE PAIN.

I'm all about finding what works… and unfortunately, a lot of the advice out there, even from trained professionals and reputable sources, *does <u>not</u> work!*

Some of the most effective methods I've discovered for eliminating pain and healing injuries are counterintuitive… and they required diligent research, testing, and creativity to discover.

People get the best results when they follow a program that's been properly designed. The best programs include only the exercises that are necessary, instructions for how to perform them properly, the proper order in which to perform them, and instructions for what the right amount of rest is and when to take it. Not doing all the steps, or performing them in the incorrect order, or taking too little rest, or too much, can throw you off course, and sometimes even make things worse!

I've learned that understanding the CAUSE of injuries and painful conditions can help heal and prevent them. For example, most people don't realize that they're doing certain things every day that put stress and tension on certain muscles, tendons, tissues and joints. Over time, this creates chronic pain and injury. Simply becoming aware, and then making tiny adjustments, can actually result in a much higher quality of life for many people.

All of my injury and exercise programs were developed as a result of my research, study and years of hands-on testing and training:

- I've been in the fitness and rehab industry since 1994.
- I spent 6 years at University studying kinesiology, corrective exercise and therapeutic exercise, and got my Master's Degree in exercise science.
- I have over 16 years of hands-on experience, working directly with clients and teaching my techniques and programs to fitness professionals, Kinesiologists, and healthcare providers.
- I've conducted thousands of personal training sessions.
- I've carefully scrutinized hundreds of relevant medical research papers.
- I'm also an author and speaker and I've given over 260 presentations to more than 5,000 fitness professionals across Canada and USA.

Rick Kaselj, MS, BSc, PK, CES
ExercisesForInjuries.com

WHAT MY CLIENTS AND CUSTOMERS SAY:

"Your exercises have changed my life. I have been in constant pain for 15 years." *Shelley Watson, Carmel, CA*

"I just wanted to say thank you for providing what I needed to resolve my hip problem! After following your exercises, I went through work all day with no pain and no pain medication. Yeah!! Thanks so much for a simple answer to a problem I have been dealing with for months." *Tracy Walker, North Carolina*

"Before I used the information, I couldn't walk normally for at least the first 15 minutes each morning. After using the program, I only have a little pain, but it eventually all got better with continued attention." *Cher Anderson, Athens, TN*

"Thank you Rick, you saved my career!" *Marco Mura, Professional Forester, Sardegna, Italy*

"I used the 90 second pain relief alone and it helped relieve the pain right away and after playing sports I feel better and the pain is not as intense. I thought I would just have to retire due to the foot pain, but I now see there is hope with your program it has helped me a lot." *Audal Acosta*

I HAVE A FREE GIFT FOR YOU...

THAT WILL START DECREASING YOUR PAIN NOW!

Before we go any further, I want to send you some of my very best stuff FOR FREE! It's my introductory gift to you. (I like to give value first, and be as helpful as I can upfront.)

My newest DVD is called "The Pain Hacker" and **I want you to have it for free.**

What is it? It's an extensive collection of 90-second pain fixes that you can do to start reducing the pain you have right now. On the video, I go through each technique slowly and carefully to show you exactly how to do them, so you can start reducing your pain and get back to a healthy, more active life.

I don't want to give away too much here, but...

- "The Pain Hacker" DVD contains 90-second pain fixes for shoulder, back, knee, elbow, foot, neck, wrist, hip, hand pain, and much more.
- The pain techniques in this DVD will work for you regardless of your current health condition, gender or age!
- With your free DVD, I'm also going to throw in two bonus programs that will teach you simple exercises that could radically change the way you feel, day-to-day.
- My unconventional "Pain Fixes" in your free DVD have been featured and talked about in these publications (and more).

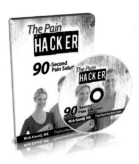

Get your FREE DVD at:
www.ThePainHacker.com/free-DVD-2

Other Products from Rick

Heal Rotator Cuff Injuries FAST

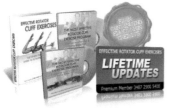
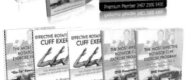

This comprehensive toolbox of 57 rotator cuff- specific exercises is EVERYTHING you need to help your clients decrease pain, improve range of motion, and increase strength in their rotator cuffs. Here are just a few of the things you'll discover:

- Why exercises that strengthen rotator cuffs do not necessarily decrease pain and increase range of motion in your clients' shoulders
- Why you shouldn't give the same exercises to every client with rotator cuff problems
- How to PROPERLY design an exercise program for the rotator cuff (I spent an entire year researching this at university, and wrote and published a paper on it in the Canadian Journal of Kinesiology)

Learn more at: www.EffectiveRotatorCuffExercises.com

Scoliosis Secrets

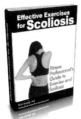
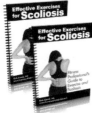
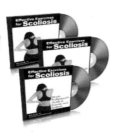

In just a few weeks, your Scoliosis patients will be thanking you! This program delivers the knowledge and exercises you need to safely and effectively train or heal anyone with Scoliosis. Here are just a few samples of what you'll learn and get in this program:

- The Three 'O' medical treatments for Scoliosis, and step–by–step instructions on how to do them
- The 7 different types of Scoliosis... how to diagnose your clients... and which exercises to prescribe for each
- CLIENT HANDOUTS that you can copy and give to your clients, completely DONE FOR YOU!

Learn more at: www.EffectiveExercisesForScoliosis.com

Scapular Stabilization Secrets

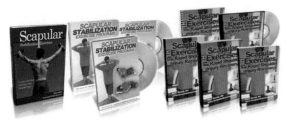

This is the RESEARCH- BACKED exercise program that will finally help your clients decrease pain, improve range of motion, and increase shoulder stability. What will you learn?

- My secret weapon for healing shoulder injuries
- Why most trainers and therapists focus on the rotator cuff in a shoulder injury, when they should focus on improving the activation, endurance, and strength of the scapular muscles
- Why your Scapular Stabilization exercise program is a waste of time... unless it includes all 5 of these components

Learn more at: www.ScapularStabilizationExercises.com

Eliminate Calf Pain (Achilles Tendinitis and Tendinosis)

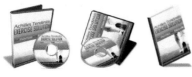
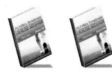

Do you have recurring pain in your calf? Have you been diagnosed with Achilles Tendinitis or Tendinosis? If so, my research -backed video exercise program is for you! Simple step–by–step videos take you through a specially -designed program to eradicate your calf pain, Achilles Tendinitis, and Tendinosis ONCE AND FOR ALL. You'll be back to hiking, walking and running before you know it. Here's a small sampling of what you'll learn in the program:

- QUICK START (non-exercise) techniques you can use to start melting your calf pain away RIGHT NOW
- ALL the exercises you need to eliminate your calf pain... AND I'll tell you the exercises that are commonly prescribed, but you don't need to worry about
- How to do each exercise, with slow, step–by–step instructions... the correct order you should follow... and how much rest you should take... to get the best and fastest results

Learn more at: www.AchillesTendinitisExercises.com

Eliminate Piriformis Syndrome

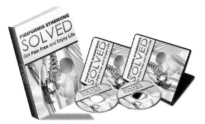

The step–by–step exercise program that ANYONE can do... that heals your Piriformis Syndrome, and allows you to: take long walks again, watch entire movies without getting up, easily lift your child... all without any pain. Here are just a few samples of what you'll learn and get in this program:

- Why you need to do more than just strengthen your core to eliminate your Piriformis Syndrome
- How to start decreasing your pain IMMEDIATELY, WITHOUT ANY EXERCISE
- These stretches and exercises are making your Piriformis Syndrome WORSE

Learn more at: www.PiriformisSyndromeSolution.com/end-piriformis-pain

Fixing Tight Hip Flexors

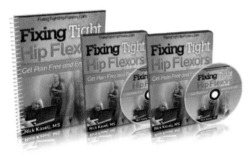

This video program has 35 exercises and other techniques designed to help you overcome painfully Tight Hip Flexors... without expensive appointments, drugs, or surgery. You'll be back to walking, running, and creating fun memories with your friends and family in just a few weeks! Here's a small sampling of what you'll learn in the program:

- THE SINGLE MOST IMPORTANT movement you need to do in order to overcome your Tight Hip Flexors (it's Component #8 in the program)
- Why it's important to decrease stress and tension in your knee, in order to fix your tight hip flexors... and how to do it properly
- The 8 CRITICAL COMPONENTS that must be included in any effective program for fixing Tight Hip Flexors (these components come from 16 years of hands–on experience and careful scrutiny of 30 separate medical research papers)

Learn more at: www.FixingTightHipFlexors.com

Heal Back Pain (Gluteus Medius Strength Program)

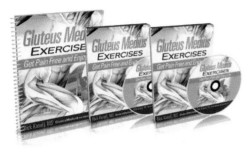

This exercise program ELIMINATES BACK PAIN by strengthening your Gluteus Medius. The Gluteus Medius is often ignored, but when properly exercised and strengthened, it can stabilize your pelvis and decrease stress on your back, which eliminates back pain. In this program, you'll learn these things (and much more):

- How to eliminate your back pain as quickly as possible (HINT: you must do the exercises in the right order so they build on each other and your progress is multiplied!)
- What most trainers and physical therapists don't know about back pain and the Gluteus Medius
- Why exercises that target your knees and hips also strengthen the Gluteus Medius and help with back pain

Learn more at: **www.GluteusMediusExercises.com**

Best Gluteus Maximus Exercises

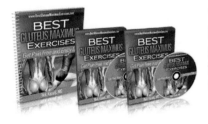

This is a fast, simple, safe, and effective program for improving your Gluteus Maximus. Most health and fitness professionals don't know about this program, or are doing it wrong. In as little as 7 days, you can go back to pain-free walking, running and living! Here are a few samples of what you'll learn in the program:

- Stretches and exercises that actually make your Gluteus Maximus WORSE
- Common mistakes people make doing Gluteus Maximus exercises
- The correct form for all of the exercises, shown step–by–step on easy–to–follow videos

Learn more at: **www.BestGluteusMaximusExercises.com**

Rick Kaselj, MS, BSc, PK, CES
ExercisesForInjuries.com

How To Speed Up Recovery Between Workouts

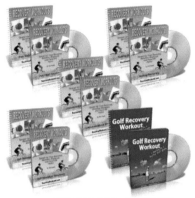

SPENDING A CENT!

Do you want to get better results from your workouts? Experience fewer aches, pains and injuries between workouts? Spend less time and money at the massage therapist? This comprehensive video program is going to help you achieve all that and more. Here are just a few of the things you'll be learning:

- What you should NEVER do if you have aches and pains between workouts
- 3 techniques and unconventional tools that RAPIDLY speed recovery between workouts
- How to get the powerful recovery effects of massage, WITHOUT

Learn more at: www.RecoveryWorkouts.com

No More Neck Pain

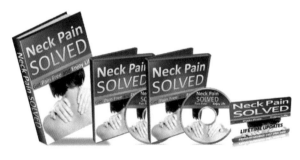

What if you could PERMANENTLY end your neck pain? This INNOVATIVE video program will teach you the simple movements and proven exercises that will make that a reality for you. Here are a few of the things you'll learn:

- An UNUSUAL technique that can start melting your neck pain away IMMEDIATELY
- How to get lasting, long- term relief for your neck... not just a temporary fix
- What I learned working with hundreds of clients with neck pain that most other professionals will never know

Learn more at: www.NeckPainSolved.com

Erase Foot & Heel Pain (Plantar Fasciitis)

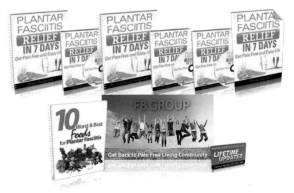

How do you eliminate Plantar Fasciitis? Do the right exercises, in the right order, with the right amount of rest. This simple, 12–week program gives you EXACTLY what you need to permanently erase your foot and heel pain. Here's a small sampling of what you'll learn:

- Why trying to strengthen your plantar fascia is a common mistake, and only makes your heel pain WORSE (hint: the plantar fascia is not a muscle!)
- One simple technique that anyone can do... that will get rid of your Plantar Fasciitis MUCH FASTER
- How to match the right exercise routine to where you are in your recovery, so you get the best results, in the least amount of time

Learn more at: www.PlantarFasciitisReliefIn7Days.com/home11

Eliminate Thoracic Outlet Syndrome

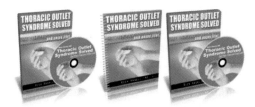

FINALLY... a simple, but effective program to overcome your Thoracic Outlet Syndrome... without expensive appointments, drugs, or surgery. My easy-to-follow, step–by–step videos and guides will help you GET PAIN- FREE in as little as 7 days. Here are just a few examples of what you'll learn in my program:

- A strange exercise I discovered using a SMALL BALL... that erased hand numbness in LESS THAN ONE MINUTE
- How to properly adjust the intensity of each exercise you do, so you can recover as quickly as possible, but also make sure you don't re-injure yourself
- The exercises you should NEVER do if you have Thoracic Outlet Syndrome

Learn more at: www.ThoracicOutletSyndromeSolved.com

Rick Kaselj, MS, BSc, PK, CES
ExercisesForInjuries.com

Eliminate Pain After Your Knee Replacement

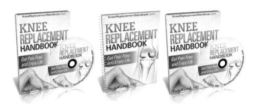

This program is perfect for getting back to a pain- free life after Knee Replacement surgery. My videos and guides give you a step–by–step program that's easy and fun to follow. You'll be back to your active and enjoyable life in just a few weeks' time. Here's a small sample of what you'll learn:

- Why my program has 9 components… and why leaving any one of them out makes it much more difficult to recover and eliminate pain
- 10 different ways you can speed up your recovery after your Knee Replacement
- Why doing exercises you find on the Internet could actually RE-INJURE YOUR KNEE

Learn more at: www.KneeReplacementHandbook.com

Overcome Your Hamstring Injury

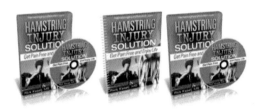

Could it really be THIS EASY to overcome your Hamstring Injury… completely on your own… without expensive physical therapy, drugs or surgery? My simple, 9–step program will erase your pain in as little as 7 days, and get you back to the full life you want. Videos, guides and photos give you the exercises and routines THAT WORK. Here's a small sampling of what you'll learn:

- Why massage isn't really helpful for Hamstring Injuries… and what is
- How to start decreasing your Hamstring pain in JUST MINUTES
- How to prevent future Hamstring Injuries

Learn more at: www.HamstringInjurySolution.com

Rick Kaselj, MS, BSc, PK, CES
ExercisesForInjuries.com

Ankle Sprain Solved

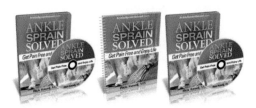

Ankle sprains are common, and mostly a minor injury. But if they aren't properly rehabilitated, they can lead to more and greater injuries. My Ankle Sprain Solved program eliminates pain and properly heals your Ankle Sprain, so you can get back to an active and engaging life. Here are a few of the things you'll learn in the program:

- How decreasing stress and tension in your knees helps heal your Ankle Sprain
- What you need to do to PERMANENTLY heal your ankle... not just get a temporary fix
- The SINGLE most important exercise you can do to heal your Ankle Sprain

Learn more at: www.AnkleSprainSolved.com

Fix Your Frozen Shoulder

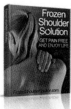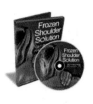

Frozen Shoulder is a common condition, but most health and fitness professionals treat it incorrectly. My program provides you with videos, guides and photos that explain this condition thoroughly, and give you a step–by–step, 7-component, 12–week program to follow that will completely eradicate your Frozen Shoulder. Here are just a few of the things you'll learn:

- The 3 most common mistakes people (and professionals) make treating Frozen Shoulder... which AGGRAVATES the condition instead of improving it
- Why stretching is an important part of fixing your Frozen Shoulder... but it's only 1 of 7 critical components in my treatment program. In my experience, the best results come when ALL 7 components are used.
- How my program is designed to provide lasting, long- term relief from Frozen Shoulder... not just a temporary fix

Learn more at: www.FrozenShoulderSolution.com

Rick Kaselj, MS, BSc, PK, CES
ExercisesForInjuries.com

Iliotibial Band (IT Band) Syndrome Solution

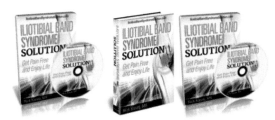

IT Band Injuries are common for runners, athletes and active people. This video -based program helps you overcome IT Band Syndrome, eliminate the pain, and get back to your active lifestyle. Here are just a few of the things you'll learn and get in this program:

- A complete program THAT ACTUALLY WORKS – it has all the exercises you need, and none that you don't
- Pain- relief techniques you can start using IMMEDIATELY
- A comprehensive explanation of how IT Band Injuries occur, and what you can do to prevent them in the future

Learn more at: www.IliotibialBandSyndromeSolution.com

Eliminate Tennis Elbow

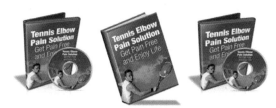

My simple, 6-step video program is PROVEN to eliminate Tennis Elbow. Before you know it, you'll once again be able to move your arms freely, pick up your kids, and grab and lift objects, all WITHOUT PAIN. Here are some of the things you'll learn in my program:

- How to diagnose yourself and make sure you definitely have Tennis Elbow
- Why you need to follow a specific plan, with a specific progression of exercises (in 3 different stages) to fully eliminate your Tennis Elbow
- How lengthening the muscles in your forearm is an important aspect of fixing your Tennis Elbow... and exactly how to do it

Learn more at: www.TennisElbowPainSolution.com

Mend Your Meniscus Tear

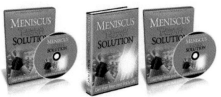

A Meniscus Tear is a nasty, painful injury... but my simple, step–by–step videos and guide will help you overcome it FAST, so you can get back to walking, running and having the active lifestyle you want. Here are just a few examples of what you'll learn in the program:

- Why a specific course of exercises and techniques is necessary to overcome your Meniscus Tear... and why you should NEVER just cobble together a random combination of exercises
- Why my program has 13 specific components, and why none of them should be left out
- The single most important movement you can do to heal your Meniscus and eliminate pain ASAP

Learn more at: www.MeniscusTearSolution.com

Lumbar Spinal Fusion Recovery Program

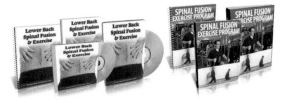

Do you have clients who are recovering from a Lumbar Spinal Fusion? I developed a special video-based exercise program for this exact situation. Video, audio and written materials give you a HIGHLY -EFFECTIVE course of treatment to get your Lumbar Spinal Fusion clients recovered QUICKLY, and give you the opportunity to earn Continuing Education Credits. Here's a tiny sampling of what you'll learn and get in the program:

- The most effective exercises for recovery from Lumbar Spinal Fusion (NOTE: most of these exercises ARE NOT taught in Personal Training Certifying Courses)
- The 5 most common reasons Lumbar Spinal Fusion surgery occurs
- A full- color HANDOUT of the EXACT Lumbar Spinal Fusion Exercise Program I give to my clients (you can print this out and give it to all your clients)

Learn more at: www.LumbarFusionExercises.com

Eliminate Sacroiliac (SI) Joint Pain FAST

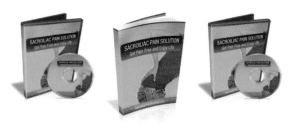

This simple, step–by–step guide will finally end your SI Joint Pain. It's a safe and effective program that most health and fitness professionals don't know about, or are doing wrong. Here are just a few of the things you'll learn:

- How Sacroiliac pain is different from regular back pain… and what to do differently to treat it
- Why doing SI Joint Pain exercises in a certain order is crucial, and what the correct order is
- The ONE movement you MUST do in order to overcome your SI Joint Pain

Learn more at: www.SacroiliacPainSolution.com/end-si-joint-pain

Eliminate Stubborn Knee Pain (Patellofemoral Syndrome)

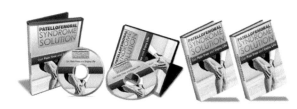

Patellofemoral Syndrome is a common condition that causes knee pain, especially for runners. Most health and fitness professionals are ineffective at treating this condition, so I created my Patellofemoral Syndrome Solution video program, which is backed by research and 16 years of hands–on experience treating thousands of people with knee pain. Here are just a few of the things you'll learn in my program:

- Why stretching DOESN'T fix Patellofemoral Syndrome
- How you can use common household items to perform all the exercises you need to ELIMINATE YOUR KNEE PAIN and get rid of Patellofemoral Syndrome FOR GOOD
- Why the order in which you do the exercises is important for success

Learn more at: www.PatellofemoralSyndromeSolution.com

Rick Kaselj, MS, BSc, PK, CES
ExercisesForInjuries.com

Shin Splints Solved

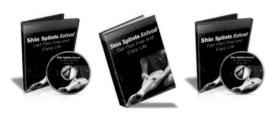

Shin Splints is a common condition, especially for runners, but most of the advice out there for treating it is ineffectual. I designed my Shin Splints Solved program after 6 years at university, 16 years of personally treating clients, and careful scrutiny of 22 relevant medical research papers. This program is HIGHLY -EFFECTIVE at eliminating Shin Splints and shin pain. You WILL be running again – without pain – before you know it! Here's just a small sample of what you'll learn in my program:

- Why ice and stretching are only temporary fixes for Shin Splints... and what to do instead to get long-lasting relief
- Why most trainers and therapists take a shotgun approach to prescribing more and more exercises, while I ask you to focus ONLY on the exercises you absolutely need (those that are most effective at eliminating Shin Splints)
- Why most health and fitness professionals don't have you strengthen your ankles... and why you MUST if you want to erase shin pain

Learn more at: www.ShinSplintsSolved.com

Jumper's Knee Solution

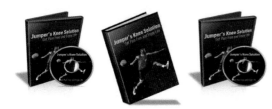

Do your knees hurt when you run or jump, especially while playing sports like basketball or volleyball? My Jumper's Knee Solution program is for you! It's a video- based exercise program that will get you back to your sports in as little as 7 days. What will you learn?

- The specific exercises that will make your pain go away FOR GOOD
- Which exercises you should NEVER do if you have Jumper's Knee
- The 10 simple steps you need to follow – IN THE CORRECT ORDER – to eliminate Jumper's Knee

Learn more at: www.JumpersKneeSolution.com

Rick Kaselj, MS, BSc, PK, CES
ExercisesForInjuries.com

Made in the USA
Charleston, SC
09 March 2017